WHAT ARE YOU WEIGHTING FOR?!

A COMPLETE WOMEN'S GUIDE TO BUILDING CONFIDENCE, STRENGTH, AND CURVES THROUGH WEIGHT TRAINING

SCOTT POWERS

CONTENTS

INTRODUCTION

Are you concerned about how you look when working out at the gym? You might constantly worry that you don't have the proper form, so you stick to cardio and leave. You struggle to understand what exercises are best for you. Maybe you've tried using the gym but stopped going after a few weeks because you didn't see the results that you wanted.

I understand your frustrations. You're not happy with the body you have because you want to be thinner, you want more muscle tone, you want to be healthier. You might want to get into bodybuilding competitions but don't know how to start training. No matter what problem you have, I have your solution in this book.

I've been weight training for over 10 years, trying extensive training programs from beginners to advanced. I have also competed in five intensive transformation programs for dropping weight and building muscle. Through my experience and determination, I've narrowed down how you can gain strength and lose weight into a simple and easy to follow guide.

First, you'll learn about the benefits of weight training. To stay motivated you need to know why this is the direction you should go and what lifting weights can do for you. I will discuss the physical, mental, and emotional gains that you will begin to feel and see.

Do you stick to the treadmill or cardio machines but wonder if there is a better exercise routine with quicker results? The answer to this is weight training. My book will help you understand how lifting weights will provide you with quicker results, burn off your unwanted fat faster, and help shape your body better than cardio.

Are you afraid of carbs? Have you tried a diet, or gone to the doctor and they explained to you that they're the root of all evil when it comes to dieting? In reality, the root of evil is unhealthy fats, though carbs can come into a close second if you find yourself sitting all day with little exercise. But this is not what you're doing. You're lifting weights, which means that carbs will become your friend instead of your enemy. The key is to eat them the right way through understanding when to have them, when not to, and how they help you develop a healthy and fit body.

Let's not forget about calories—another word that many people fear while trying to lose weight. Don't be afraid of eating calories; they're necessary when you're working out because you're burning more energy and boosting your metabolism. But you do want to count your calories, and I will help you do this without needing to give up your favorite foods or completely restrict yourself. I'll teach you how to find the right balance of carbs for your lifestyle so you can maintain a healthy weight.

It's time to let go of the embarrassment you feel when you're working out in front of other people. I will help you feel empowered when lifting weights at the gym. You will no longer worry about anyone judging your exercising form or body. I will not only discuss proper form but also give you tips to help you overcome your feelings of being watched and judged.

The training I provide in this book focuses on developing tone in your upper and lower body. You'll discover the easiest workouts for your problem areas, whether it's your arms, abs, back, calves, or glutes. Not only will you learn different exercises, but you'll understand the anatomy of your body parts and how these workouts will give you the curves that you desire.

I know you're wondering about those moments where you can't get to your fitness center or you just don't feel like heading to the gym. My guide will help you build toned muscle at home without weights. You will learn two full body workouts that will describe the exercises and how to do them with proper form.

Let's not forget about the key of consistency. It takes time to develop a habit and get into an exercise routine, so I want to help you stay motivated by providing you with tips and ways to help maintain consistency so you achieve your desired results.

I'm not just writing this book because of my experience. I'm doing it because of my passion to help you find the easiest path to lose weight and build strength. I want to teach you how to stay motivated so you can keep the body you want. I will help you build your self-confidence, so you walk into the gym like you own it. Assisting you in your weight training goals matters deeply to me because the skills and methods you learn in this book helped myself, family, and friends reach their desired weight and physical strength.

You're not on this journey alone. Start building your new and healthier lifestyle by turning to the next chapter with me so you can learn about the five biggest benefits to weight lifting.

THE FIVE BIGGEST BENEFITS OF WEIGHT TRAINING FOR WOMEN

One of the biggest challenges when it comes to weight training is self-motivation. First, it's not easy to change your daily routine, which may consist of cardio only, several days a week. Second, on average it takes about 21 days to get into a new routine. Third, you want to see results right away but this isn't always possible with cardio exercise only. You might also be ashamed or feel embarrassed to walk into the gym if you haven't been exercising regularly and you see toned bodies all around you. You may worry what people will say about you, to you, or even wonder if the two women in the back are laughing at you. It's hard to stay motivated when you're not comfortable with where you're going and what you're doing.

It's important that I start you on this process by telling you about the five biggest benefits of weight training for you. Yes, there are many other benefits that I won't cover in-depth, but I wanted to focus on five things because they're the biggest ways to push yourself into starting weight training or going back to it.

As you build about confidence, learn about building curves in the right areas, and other benefits, imagine yourself seeing these results. Don't just read the words, but visualize yourself noticing your new curves, getting that slimmer waistline, buying new clothes, and feeling less anxious. For example, close your eyes and see yourself looking in a full-length mirror and notice how your hourglass shape is forming. You're comparing your new body to the body you had several months ago. You're noticing amazing changes and you feel better. You feel like you have more energy one weight at the time. Taking the time to think about how these benefits will make you feel as you start your journey will only increase your motivation. You can bring yourself back to your visualization and emotions you felt in this moment when you're struggling to get up in the morning for your workout.

BOOST SELF-CONFIDENCE

The changes in your physique are important when you start lifting weights, but what happens on the inside is just as important. In fact, you might see it as more important because it can help you improve all areas of your life, especially when it comes to your self-confidence.

Jessie Hilgenberg is a fitness model, IFBB Figure Pro, figure and bikini competition coach, and NLA Performance sponsored athlete who inspires women to become their best selves through her workout plans which focus on lifting. She uses her personal experience to show you that you can achieve everything in your power once you start to boost your confidence. Instead of walking into the gym and standing beside your partner or friend when working out because you're worried about what people think when they look at you, you'll walk into the gym like you own it. You won't worry about what others are thinking because you'll know they are focused on your proper form. You'll feel that they're watching you so they can practice in the same way. In fact, you'll have people who come up to you asking for advice and tips.

Not only will you have people telling you how good you look, but you will believe it because you emotionally, physically, and mentally feel it. Lifting weight increases energy and makes you feel happier and healthier. When you feel better on the inside, you feel better about your outside appearance. Your mindset changes from wanting to hide in the corner while working out to standing in the center.

Exercising, especially weight training, is challenging. You find yourself feeling pushed to your limits but you don't give up. You focus on what you can do in that moment and then you set your goal. You strive to reach that goal every day you're working out and this helps you overcome any physical or mental challenges you face. You will feel that training is rewarding you by constantly proving your power and ability. The key is to lift weights in a self-disciplined and correct manner, by setting your routine and sticking with it, including a healthy diet. You will also want to ensure you understand the correct form and know any signs your body gives that you're pushing yourself too much and need to progress at a slower pace.

Not everyone needs to lose weight, but for those of you who do, losing weight will also improve your confidence because you're focusing on eating healthy, you feel better physically, mentally, and emotionally. It's important to note that all of these factors work closely together to form your overall well-being . For example, when you're feeling happy and confident, you're more likely to focus on eating healthy. Weight training will also lower your risk of diabetes, prevent back pain, regulate blood glucose levels, help to fight osteoporosis, and protect the health of your heart—all of which increases your overall health.

Boosting your confidence becomes a ripple effect, going deeper than improving your gym life. This means that you'll feel better working out, at home, work, and everywhere else. You will feel your best under stress, perform at your potential. Leadership becomes easier when you feel confident and people will start to see you as an inspiration and you'll feel valued. You will feel happier in your life overall.

BURN MORE CALORIES AND FAT

Some of the main reasons you may turn to exercise is to lose weight, gain muscle, or have a toned, proportional body. Burning calories is the key to weight loss. At first, you probably thought that you need to run, walk several times a day, or hit the gym to focus on cardio exercises to lose weight quickly. But, one of the best ways to burn calories is through weight training because it requires more energy, which means you need more calories to burn than you're used to.

There are two types of exercise, anaerobic (weight lifting) and aerobic (cardio). When you focus on the first, you have low duration and high intensity where the second has low intensity and high duration. This means you can focus on cardio exercises for a longer time because you don't need to put as much energy into them and you get the oxygen you need. Of course, the faster you run the more this changes, but unless you're training for the Olympics or a race you usually don't run too fast, which can turn into high intensity.

When you flip the switch to anaerobic, you don't get as much oxygen into your body. This means your body starts burning sugars from your cells to help you get the oxygen your body needs. It also means that you don't exercise as long because you need to catch your breath. Because you don't work as long, people think that anaerobic isn't as effective when burning calories, but it's more effective because you start to break down sugars.

The Certified Strength and Conditioning Specialist (CSCS) and a National Strength and Conditioning Association-Certified Personal Trainer (NSCA-CPT) of Rocky's Fitness Center, located in Santa Cruz, CA, states it best: "Immediately following a strength training session, the body needs to replenish the energy drained and repair the muscle damage that has been caused...The repair process uses aerobic energy for several hours" Schaefer (2015).

You will also burn more calories because your muscles grow. It is recommended that you have between 1,500 and 1,600 calories a day at minimum, meaning you can eat more. Think of it this way—for every pound of muscle you have, you need between six to ten calories every day for it to maintain itself. The more you lift weight, the higher this number goes. This also means that you need to focus on the right areas and switch up your routine at times. You need to understand what weight lifting techniques will give you the biggest gain for the curves you want. The best exercises to try so you don't increase your weight but your muscle tone are lunges, pull-ups, push-ups, squats, and deadlifts. All of these exercises will be discussed in later chapters so you learn proper form for the best results.

Another reason you need to count your calories is because your metabolism increases with weight lifting, including after your workout. Therefore, your body needs more calories as it will burn more of them. But, you also need to think of the whole 24-hour period. That's right, you also need to eat the right amount of calories so your body can continue to burn its fuel when you're sleeping. Your body needs calories around the clock so you need to do what you can to ensure you are consuming the calories you need to sustain you for a 24-hour period.

BUILD CURVES IN THE RIGHT AREAS

There are curves that you want to show off and then there are places on your body where you'd rather not see curves. I know you know the areas I'm talking about. You want that hourglass figure with the small waist, curvy hips, and strong shoulders. Don't be embarrassed about it because it happens to nearly everyone. You're looking in the mirror one day and you notice something and think, "Wait a minute, where did this curve come from?" If this sounds like a part of your life and you're ready to change, it's time to look at weight training because you'll be able to focus on those target areas and shape your legs, shoulders, back, glutes, arms, core, and many other areas.

Personal trainers will agree with me, one of the best ways to get the figure you want it by weight lifting. Exercise specialist and personal trainer Liz Letchford states, "Heavy lifting is the best way to create strong, curvy hips and a tiny waist" (Florio, 2018). This is because adding muscle to your figure helps define the feminine body.

The key is to know where to begin, and you need to look at more than where you want to build your curves. You need to have the right routine for you, including taking short breaks to rest. If you know you want to focus on your hip area, it's a good idea to start here because this can give you a psychological motivator to continue with your training. It's one of the areas that you can see the best results the quickest, especially if you follow proper form.

Another key is to not forget about your upper body. There seems to be a theme on social media that states you should focus on your glutes to get the booty that you want. While this is important, to get the best figure overall, you need to focus on your chest, shoulders, and upper back. One way to do this is by switching your exercise routine. You can focus on your glutes three days and your upper routine the other two days.

You also need to look at the amount of weights you're lifting. It's tempting to try the lighter bars, the ones you know that you can safely handle. But, this won't give you the intensity that you need to burn those carbs and lose body fat. You want to focus on the heavier weights, working up to them so you don't damage your muscle and push yourself.

To help give you an idea of where to start, if you don't hire a personal trainer, Letchford says to keep it random. You want to focus on your heavy lifting on one body area per week. For example, you work on squats on Monday, push-ups on Tuesday, and then deadlifts on Wednesday. You can then look at pull-ups for Thursday and maybe mix it up on Friday with your favorites.

Another benefit of having curves exactly where you want them is the clothes you get to buy. Did I just tell you to go out and buy a whole new closet? Well, no, not really, but you will need to purchase a few more items for your closet. You can go for the look you've been wanting to try but felt that your body wasn't right for it. Soon, that little black dress, yoga pants and skinny jeans can be a regular part of your wardrobe, including a special tank top that will show off your shoulder, upper back, and arm muscles.

THE FOUNTAIN OF YOUTH: STAY YOUNGER, LONGER

You've heard about it before—the fountain of youth. It's an idea that you've probably wished was true as you were blowing at your birthday candles. The reality is, there is a fountain of youth and that's weight training. While it can't cut down on your actual age, it can help you strengthen bones. As you age, you tend to focus less on exercises and movement. You retire, you start to ache due to arthritis and other health issues, and you lose energy faster. This increases if you don't take the time to exercise and focus on a healthy diet from a young age. In fact, your lack of activity and poor diet can take about 1% of your bone mass every year after the age of 40. Brittle bones lead to fractures, breaks, and more health problems.

Weight lifting also helps prevent osteoporosis, which is another concern as you age. While about two million men have the condition, over eight million women are diagnosed in the United States (Harvard Health Publishing, 2019). You want to decrease your chances of this bone disease because it's one of the leading causes of fractures, especially in the hip. Harvard Health states that six out of every ten people will not regain their previous level of independence after a hip fracture. It can easily lead you into early entry in long-term care facilities because you'll struggle with walking short distances.

Studies show that strength training will not only decrease osteoporosis, but it can even help build a new bone. When you show signs of the disease, your new bones have trouble keeping up with the removal of the old bones, which causes them to become brittle and even form holes. You won't realize you have this health problem until you fall or walk and your bones simply break. When you start lifting weights, your new bones can keep up with the old ones and repair any damage, making them stronger for a longer period of time. One study shows that by the time women reach 70 years old, they've lost about 50% of their muscle mass unless they've started weight lifting. It won't help keep all of the muscle mass as you naturally lose some when you age, but it can help decrease the amount you lose. It works because you tend to target the bones and muscles that become weakest as you age, which is your arms, shoulders, hips, spine, and wrists. Whatever age you are, it's never too late to start weight training to improve your overall health and bones and muscle.

REDUCE STRESS AND ANXIETY

You've been there at some point in your life or you're there now —struggling with anxiety and stress. You might feel that the last few months have been worse or bring yourself back to a time where you felt trapped. You didn't believe that you would make something of your life. You couldn't handle the pressure of working full-time, taking care of a family, and paying bills. It's okay to admit that stress and anxiety feel like chains holding you back from becoming your best self. The key is to not let yourself stay in that mindset. Finding a hobby that can reduce the stress you have in your life may help you control your anxiety.

What better way to start this new path than with weight training? You've already learned about four out of the five benefits. Now, it's time to dive into one of the most common benefits that will help you change your life around. You don't just need to depend on other weight-lifters who say that it helps their mental health, you can also look at the studies proving that lifting weights will help ease your worries, fears, and stress of daily life.

Sports Medicine published a study in 2017 that showed weight training helped people reduce their symptoms of anxiety. *JAMA Psychiatry* followed through on this study and further stated that not only will it decrease your worries and fears but also can prevent depression (Stulberg, 2018).

Researchers state there are many reasons why this happens. First, exercise lifts your mood. It makes you feel confident and empowered, which is why many women lift weights in the morning. It gives them the mindset they need at work, especially if they are a part of a male-dominated field.

Another benefit to weight lifting is improved sleep. Working out takes more energy and gives you an easier night's rest, especially during the moments before you fall asleep. It's usually during this time, especially for women, that you stay up late worrying about everything you didn't do today or need to do tomorrow. You might even start to think about the mistakes you made years ago. The trouble is, the less sleep you get, the more worry and anxiety pervade your thoughts.

You may also start to see your anxiety deescalating because your self-confidence improves. Once you gain more confidence, your self-worth begins to increase. You know your worth, where your strengths are, and no one can tell you differently because you believe in yourself.

Psychologists see weight training as a form of exposure therapy, meaning you face your fears head-on. While you probably didn't directly fear lifting weights, you did have some fears about it. Working toward increasing the weight through your workouts can help you realize that you can overcome obstacles.

It can improve your motivation to try new directions in life, knowing that you can overcome any obstacles in front of you. For instance, you might have a fear of going back to school because you don't know if you can manage your time. After a few weeks of weight training, you might feel that you can go back to school because you know you can get help from your family and learn time management.

Finally, your anxiety and stress will decrease because you look at the world in a different way. You can feel more positive and this helps you see the world in a brighter light. For example, instead of telling yourself, "I can't do this, I'm not smart or good enough," you'll say, "I can accomplish this with hard work and dedication." In a sense, you'll start to switch your thoughts, elevating your self-confidence and self-worth.

2

WEIGHT TRAINING VS CARDIO

There is a relationship between strength training and cardio that many people don't know about. For years, probably closer to a couple of decades, people have looked at the difference and similarities to try to tell other people which exercise routine will be best for them. The debate tends to go back and forth and sometimes it depends on who you talk to, such as your physician or what trainer you train with in the gym. You might have, or develop, certain health conditions that make you look at the benefit of strength training over cardio. For example, if you have heart disease you will be pushed towards cardio and while this is a great routine for you, it doesn't mean that you should forget about lifting weights. You just need to stay within your restrictions.

BENEFITS OF CARDIO AND WEIGHTLIFTING

The key to knowing which is better for you or how to build the perfect relationship for your health and body is to understand them separately so you can place them together. You already know five of the best benefits for weight lifting, so now it's time to look at cardio's benefits.

Regulate appetite. One of the biggest challenges when you're trying to lose weight is sticking with your diet. It's hard to know what you should and should not eat when you're focusing on a certain exercise routine and you're not sure how to start with the research or who to talk to. While you know that you need more calories to burn with strength training, you also need to understand how a cardiovascular workout will influence your appetite.

You're lifting weight regularly and you've felt an increase in hunger, especially during your exercise time. This is common because you need the energy you gain from the foods you eat to keep your body going during and after an intense weight lifting routine. But, when you combine your routine with high-intensity cardio, such as cycling or moderate-pace running, you're going to curb your appetite because you get your blood flowing around your body instead of just in your stomach area. You'll start to feel yourself slowly losing weight with cardio, especially if you tend to stress eat or overeat in general. You'll feel less hungry and as long as you follow your diet and only eat when you're hungry, you'll see results quickly.

Improves heart health. One of the main reasons people turn to cardio, and also ignore weight training, is the benefit to their heart. When you have poor circulation or cardiovascular conditions, you can improve your heart's health through certain exercises. It will help your heart pump blood and work easily, especially when it's put under pressure. It's important to note that the earlier you begin the better condition your heart will be.

If you're a jogger, you've noticed how it's become easier over time. In fact, you might remember feeling like you were going to pass out when you went for a run the first time. This is because your heart couldn't keep up the pumping. You probably felt like it was about to beat out of your chest. But, by the time you went out for your fifth or sixth jog, you noticed your breathing was better, you could go for a longer period of time, and your heart doesn't seem to beat as wildly as it did before. This is because your ticker is pumping more efficiently as blood is flowing throughout your body.

Aids your immune system. One of the main ways for you to stay healthy is to take care of your immune system. For example, studies prove that people who struggle with depression find themselves physically sick often, catching the flu even after receiving the flu shot or they will battle the common cold. It's especially important now to protect your immune system because there are a lot of new diseases, such as COVID-19.

Fortunately, adding cardio to your weekly routine will improve your body so your immune system can fight off the unwanted bacteria and viruses without you feeling sick. This happens because moderate exercise increases the immunoglobulines, which are molecules in your system that help fight off disease.

Boost brain power. It happens to everyone—you're in the grocery store and looking everywhere for your list but can't find it. You do your best to purchase the food you need by memory and then get home to see you forgot your shopping list on your table. Cognitive performance starts to decline around the age of 30. What this means is you don't need to feel bad when you walk into your kitchen and forget why you're there. You're not alone.

The positive note is that research focusing on cardiovascular exercise proves that you'll improve the functions of your brain by reducing the amount of lost brain tissue over time. This means that your memory will stay sharp, you'll be more mindful, and you'll decrease your chances of cognitive disorders later in life, if you keep up with your workout routine on a consistent basis. Plus, by adding a little bit of cardio into your weight training routine, you'll strengthen the fountain of youth.

Hearing that you have high blood pressure from your doctor is usually cause for concern at any age. The biggest problem for the health field is that younger people are entering their doors with hypertension or high blood pressure. While the younger generation doesn't worry too much about it, physicians are looking at ways to decrease these statistics because of the dangers it creates. For example, you're at a higher risk of heart disease and stroke, damage to your blood vessels, and potentially death.

Typically, you need to make a lot of lifestyle changes to lower your blood pressure, such as stopping smoking, cutting out caffeine, reducing stress, increasing exercise, eating a healthy diet, and losing extra pounds. Fortunately, you can reach several of these changes by simply following cardio and focusing on a better diet. Another benefit is you can usually lower your blood pressure without having to add medication to your daily routine.

Reduces chronic pain. It seems that the older you get, the more pain you feel every day. I would say if you're not feeling chronic pain yet, just wait, but you can also decrease it by adding cardio (and weight lifting) to your exercise regimen. It's known to lower pain associated with your upper body, specifically your back, when you focus on low aerobic exercises like swimming. Part of this is because cardio helps decrease the inflammation in your body, which causes the pain.

Helps you sleep. One factor you might notice is that cardio and weight lifting have a lot of the same benefits and one is better sleep. A study completed by colleagues at Northwestern

University in Chicago, Illinois, studied several participants for 16 weeks. They focused on aerobic activities and completed questionnaires focusing on their mood and sleep. All of the participants claimed they had insomnia prior to the study. For the duration, they completed a daily cardio exercise program and learned about sleep hygiene. The researchers concluded that while exercising within two hours before going to bed didn't help the participants sleep, completing their routine earlier in the day helped them fall asleep faster and stay asleep during the night. Participants also recorded that they feel better throughout the day because they had more energy (Reid et al., 2010).

Budget friendly. Exercising is not always easy on your pocketbook, especially if you want to purchase all the equipment for your home gym or you have to spend a large amount of money on a specific gym membership or personal trainer. One benefit of both cardio and weight lifting is that you can have a budget that fits your needs and finances. There are a lot of high-intensity workouts that you can do at home or outside for free. The biggest factor here is getting yourself motivated and setting aside time to ensure you get your routine in before the end of the day.

A FITNESS FACEOFF

Through the benefits of cardio and weight lifting, you know that combining them can give you the best results. You will also notice that when one exercise routine lacks the benefit you are looking for in a certain area, the other will help strengthen it. In other words, they can sometimes balance each other out if used correctly. In this case, you need to understand more than just the benefits and try to match your routine to get the best flow. You need to create the perfect workout that will give you the best curves. Let's break it down by looking at it section by section.

What is the best routine to take and keep off your excess pounds?

It's estimated that you'll burn between 10 to 12 calories every minute that you use high-intensity cardio exercises, such as running and cycling. When you compare this to the 8 to 10 calories that you can burn when you lift weights every minute, you might feel that the winner is cardio, but you need to look a bit deeper.

When you focus on cardio, you don't get the metabolic spike after your workout. Your body doesn't need to focus on recovering your muscles, so you'll start to burn calories slowly after ending your routine. Therefore, you end up burning more calories through weight lifting because you have to add in the additional 20% to 25% that you'll burn off after your workout.

So, the winner when it comes to taking off excess pounds is— strength training!

What is the best routine to improve your self-confidence?

If you follow both training programs, you'll notice that you feel better about yourself whether you've finished running or lifting weights. In fact, if you look at professional weight lifters or swimmers, they all show high confidence in their abilities. This can make you assume that either routine will improve the way you feel about yourself. While this is true, one will give you stronger self-confidence than the other.

When you cross the finish line after a race, you feel good about yourself. You feel like you accomplished a task and this gives you motivation to run the following year and continue your workout. It doesn't matter if you finished last, the point is that you finished. The problem with your confidence is if you don't follow through with another race or continue to consistently follow an aerobic training routine, your confidence will start to fade. It's also possible that you only feel good about yourself for a short period of time.

You look in the mirror as you finish lifting weights for 20 minutes and believe that you look good. Looking closely at your arms and legs, they seem more toned and this increases your confidence. Researchers have looked into this inflated self-image by studying women who gave surveys about their self-confidence and views of their body when they started lifting weights and 12 weeks after the program. Not only did it show their appearance changed, but it showed significant change when it came to their self-esteem. They wanted to continue working out because they not only saw results but also felt them.

The winner for which routine is the best to strengthen your confidence is (drum roll please) strength training!

What strategy will help you relieve the most stress?

Scientific researchers have studied the stress relief benefits of cardio for longer than those of weight lifting. So far, cardio has the lead. In 2005, the *European Journal of Sports Science* concluded in a study that focusing on cardio exercises, such as swimming and playing tennis, for 15 minutes two to three times a week reduces anxiety significantly (Plosser, 2007). You can further increase these statistics to 50% by exercising three to five days a week.

Cardio gives you meditation in motion. When you're focusing on a game or your routine, you forget about the problems you're facing or unanswered questions you have. You don't think about what you need to do and what you don't. Instead, your mind is concentrating on your movements. But, the same can be said about weight training. You're focused on your form and how much weight you're pushing or pulling.

The "feel good" neurotransmitters known as endorphins are released when you're physically active. Even though many people refer to this as a "runner's high," it doesn't matter what routine you're following. You'll release them during any intense workout from lifting weight to swimming. Endorphins also help your mental health because they make you realize that the problems you felt were huge mountains to climb are really small hills you can easily scale. You look at the world through a different set of lenses. Instead of standing in the middle of the issue and seeing it all around, you bring yourself up and look down to see its true size.

The winner for this round of fitness faceoff is cardio and weight training! Even though lifting weights is a bit behind scientifically, the results are starting to match cardio's benefits.

What is the best exercise routine to follow when you want to limit sprains, stress fractures, etc.?

One of the challenges of exercises, no matter what strategy you follow, is that you need to pay attention to what you're doing. You have to listen to your body so you don't cause any internal damage that can make you sit on the sidelines.

Cardio focuses on repetitive movements during most of the training exercises, whether it's tennis, racketball, or running. You can take a break from some of the pressure on your knees and ankles if you mix your routine with swimming, but this isn't possible for many people. The cartilage between your bones, tendons, muscles, joints, and ligaments takes a lot of stress, which can develop weak points if you don't exercise correctly.

Weight lifting also places pressure when you repeat your routine every day, but you're able to change it up more easily between your upper and lower body. You can also strengthen your muscles, bones, and everything in between with lifting. By focusing on certain aspects of your body that are weaker, such as ankles, you can build them up so they don't break or fracture easily. Senior athletic trainer and research coordinator at the University of Wisconsin-Madison, Tim McGuine states, "Functional strength training teaches your brain to allow muscle contractions that are quick enough to prevent or minimize injuries" (Plosser, 2007).

What all this information tells you when it comes to this round is that weight lifting in the winner!

What routine should you incorporate if you want to win the next community race?

You might think that the automatic winner is cardio. It's a safe assessment because you can practice running and speed. For example, if you want to participate in a swim meet, you need to learn to breathe underwater and pace yourself. If you want to join the 5k race for charity, you need to learn how to focus on speed and endurance for the best results.

You should never ignore strength training to boost your speed because lifting weights will improve your stride power. But, you need to focus on the right training regimen, such as the standing triple jump which is when you swing your arms back, jump forward in a leap, land on your right foot, and jump between your left and right foot a few times. You can repeat this repetition for 10 to 12 reps or for three to five minutes.

So, which routine wins the race? The answer is both. Professionals state if you want the best chance of strengthening your stride, you'll mix cardio and weight lifting into your plan.

Which routine should you use if you want to add years to your life?

The key to growing old is to take care of your body. This means that you will want to decrease your chances of heart disease and other illnesses. You will also want to keep your weight to a healthy number and follow the right diet.

You know that weight training will help you shed those pounds and keep them off. You can schedule two sessions every week to decrease the amount of intra-abdominal fat in your body, which is the fat that constricts blood vessels and wraps around your organs. A consistent schedule will help you keep an unhealthy level of this fat out of your body, adding more years to your lifespan.

Cardio will also help you celebrate more birthdays because it reduces the risk of diabetes, heart disease, osteoporosis, stroke, obesity, and even some cancers. The more you sweat, the bigger the benefits as a strong heart will pump more blood with each beat. Furthermore, you can prevent internal inflammation that can cause you to become ill quickly with anything from the common cold to cancer. It will also decrease your chances of arthritis.

So, which should be your best friend at the gym? According to science the winner is cardio because there are more studies to support this theory when looking at longevity. However, weight training comes in at a close second.

When you combine cardio with weight training, you can spend less time on the dreaded cardio equipment because weight training will boost metabolism far after you have finished working out. You can create variety for your exercise routines by focusing on lifting a few days of the week and cardio for the other days. Both will also give you the added bonus of feeling better overall, whether you're looking at your physical, mental, emotional, or even spiritual health. You will gain the best curves that you can by mixing these routines and maintaining the best diet for you.

3

FALL IN LOVE WITH CARBS AGAIN

You've heard so many times, whether it was from a doctor, friend, or the media, "You need to cut down your carbs in order to lose weight." You have probably heard it so many times that you've tried several times to follow the regular 2,000 calorie diet or even go down to half of that. The trouble with calories is that your body is used to a certain amount, so when you suddenly decrease it you will end up with cravings that you can't ignore. You might start to crave carbs or sugar because you are cutting back on those foods. Then, you have those television commercials that always advertise the worst foods for your body but look so good in your mind. When you're craving certain nutrients in your foods, such as iron or protein, you'll start to find fast food appetizing because your mind associates the hamburger to protein. So what happens? You go into your kitchen and have a late night snack because it's hard to sleep when you're hungry.

Lifting weights can help you with the cravings because its intensity requires fuel. You will need to eat carbohydrates to sustain your energy before workouts and afterwards for muscle recovery. Am I basically saying that you can eat more carbs than you realize when weight training? Possibly; it depends on how many you're thinking about. There is a magic number and it often depends on how long you work out and the intensity of your routine. The reality is, your body needs carbohydrates to grow and maintain muscle. Dieting can be made simple when lifting weights because you will be burning more calories and fat. You can be less strict and stingy and still obtain great results if lifting with intensity.

WEIGHT LIFTING AND YOUR BASIC NUTRITION

One key is to ensure you focus on the essential macronutrients so you can keep your cells healthy while building muscle and receiving energy. Macronutrients are often called macros and include protein, carbohydrates, and fat. You also need micronutrients which are vitamins and minerals. However, these are taken in smaller amounts. When you find a healthy balance, especially of macros, your body can decrease fat, maintain lean tissue, and repair muscles. When you lift weights, you essentially create microscopic tears in your connective tissue and muscle fibers. If you don't repair them through nutrients, they won't heal correctly and become more prone to damage. You could also suffer with muscle pain and problems throughout the rest of your life. Another reason to eat balanced nutrients is because you will also feel better when you're heading to the gym, which can give you motivation to continue your schedule.

One basic rule is to eat 0.5 to 1 gram of protein per pound you weigh or 1.2 to 2 grams of protein per kilogram of weight. For example, if you weigh 150 pounds, you will want to eat at least 75 to 100 grams of protein every day. If you weigh 100 kilograms, you'll want to eat 120 to 200 grams. You might feel that this sounds like more protein than you planned on eating during the day. People are usually surprised by the grams of protein they need to consume, but it's necessary and easier to find than you think. For example, by eating three ounces of cooked, lean chicken breast you get 27 grams of protein, one cup of cooked quinoa is eight grams, one cup of cooked chickpeas is 15 grams, and one seven ounce container of nonfat Greek yogurt is 17 grams (Corleone, 2020). Another reason to ensure you eat the right amount of protein is it will help you stay full for longer. This will help curb your cravings, give you more energy, help you fall asleep faster, and aid in digestion.

When it comes to carbohydrates, you want to eat about 6 to 10 per kilogram of weight or 2.7 to 4.5 grams per pound of body weight. For example, if you weigh 75 kilograms, you will want to consume 450 to 750 carbs in your daily diet. If you're 175 pounds, you will ensure you eat 472.5 to 787.5 carbs. If you're struggling to learn how many calories you should eat because you're increasing your activity gradually or would just need some guidance, there are several online calorie calculators that can give you a start. All you need to do is answer a few questions, such as your gender, weight, height, and your activity level. Another way to calculate your carbs is to think of the amount of calories you consume. The National Academies of Sciences, Engineering and Medicine states that carbohydrates should include 45 to 65% of your calorie intake (Corleone, 2020).

When it comes to fat intake, you don't need to focus on a specific number, but you want to be aware of how much you consume. It's best to focus on healthy fats or plant-based foods for your diet. Healthy or "good" fats are unsaturated while the "bad" is also known as trans fats. For example, the fat you'll eat in a fast-food burger is trans while the fat you get in fish, seeds, sunflower oil, olive oil, and nuts are unsaturated. There are also saturated fats that aren't as unhealthy as trans fats but they're also not as healthy as unsaturated. You can eat more of these foods than you can trans fat foods, but you should limit them to a certain amount every day or week. These foods include cheese, milk, red meat, and butter. You can also turn to the National Academies of Sciences, Engineering and Medicine which guides you to get 20 to 35% of your calories from fat.

Another key is to know when you should eat macros. That's right, you don't just want to run to them whenever you hear your stomach grumble. Instead, you want to tie your meals into your exercise regimen so you can receive the best benefits with lifting and your diet. For example, recent scientific research shows that eating during certain times around your workout can help improve your mood, give you more energy, and enhance recovery with tissue and muscles (Kerksick et al., 2008).

The first step to focusing on when to eat is to think of your calories Even though they are seen as the evil twin of a diet, they can help you stay healthy. You want to eat a certain amount every day, but you don't want to eat the majority of them in one meal. This can easily happen if you focus on higher calories during dinner time, whether you're working out during this time or not. The best step to take is to follow the USDA 2015-2020 Dietary Guidelines, which states women who strength train regularly should consume between 2,000 to 2,400 calories daily. If you need to adjust your calories, you should do so gradually through 50 to 100 increments. For example, if you realize that you eat 2,700 calories and you should be closer to 2,300, start by decreasing 50 calories every day. After a couple of days you can decrease another 50 to 100. You can also consult your primary care physician to help you find the best balance and how you should decrease according to your weight lifting goals and health.

You also want to meet your calorie intake because if you're lacking them, your muscles and tissues can't repair themselves and this will affect your training. It can also make you more tired or harder to fight off your cravings. You can start to struggle mentally because you can't concentrate and problem-solving skills decline when you don't have enough energy for brain power. If you continue to eat fewer calories than you should, your health can continue to decline which will further cause problems with weight training. Fortunately, once you figure out how many calories you should consume every day, you can download an app to your phone to track your calories.

WHAT YOU SHOULD EAT BEFORE YOU START WEIGHT TRAINING

When you talk to athletes and professional trainers, they will tell you that one of the most important meals of your day is your pre-workout meal. It will help you improve your performance and keep you more mindful when it comes to your form. In return, you'll feel the benefits sooner and recover from your training faster. Plus, it's not good to exercise on an empty stomach because you'll lose energy quickly, get a headache, develop abdominal pains, and you can pass out.

The best time to consume your meal is between 60 to 90 minutes before you begin your workout. However, if your stomach needs to settle a little more because you start to feel nauseous, you can try eating about two hours before you start exercising. If you still have problems with your training, then eat sooner. You can find your best time by increasing the time between eating and working out by 15 to 30 minute increments each time. Some people find that their optimal time is four hours while others are closer to two.

You should try to consume about the same amount of protein and carbohydrates. You want to keep it between 30 to 45 grams. So, if you eat 35 grams of carbs you want to eat around 35 grams of protein. Don't just guess that amount of grams you should eat because it goes by your body type. For instance, if you're overweight you want to eat closer to 45 grams where someone who is smaller will reduce their amount. As an example, you can choose to eat one whole egg mixed with three egg whites and two slices of whole wheat bread for a larger meal whereas a smaller serving will include half that or one cup of cottage cheese and one banana. You can also add a few unsaturated fats to help create a stronger balance, such as nuts or seeds.

But, what happens if you're rushing or life throws off your routine and you can't eat at your normal time? You find yourself starving by the time you're heading to the gym and start to wonder if you should skip your workout, move it to a later time, or skip your meal. The best answer is none of these. Instead, you want to eat a lighter meal and keep your workout consistent. For instance, if you eat between 40 to 45 grams of carbs and protein, decrease it to 20 to 30 grams, especially if you have stomach issues when you eat close to working out. If you're about 15 to 30 minutes away from hitting the gym, choose a light snack of about 10 to 20 grams instead of a light meal.

If you eat about four hours ahead of training, some of the best foods to enjoy are energy bars, yogurt, bagels, fresh fruit, pasta with tomato sauce, cereal with milk, baked potato, and whole wheat toast with peanut butter, lean meat, or cheese.

Eating two to three hours ahead includes oatmeal, fresh fruit, bagel, whole wheat pasta, Greek yogurt, and whole wheat bread.

Some of the best foods to eat within an hour before you start exercising are fresh fruit or half a cup of a sports drink.

Now that you have an idea of the best foods, you need to know what items to stay away from. Of course, they're usually known as the "goodies" in many homes but it's essential to refrain from quickly grabbing them for your breakfast because it can hurt you more than help you down the road. Foods you shouldn't touch include ones with a lot of fiber and unhealthy fats, such as potato chips, donuts, fried foods, red meat, and candy bars—in general, any foods that are hard to digest. The main reason for this is not just because they're bad for you but they can cause stomach cramps and make you feel emotionally, mentally, and physically drained. You might explain it as exhaustion or slug-gishness. If you tend to have intestinal issues, it's also a good idea to stay away from beans, dairy, and dried fruit as they can make you gassy during your workout. While it happens to everyone, you probably don't want to have this issue or need to run to a public restroom in the middle of your training session. It's just best to spare yourself from this type of potential awkwardness.

It's also important to remember your fluids. You especially want to ensure you drink enough water but sports drinks are also a viable choice. While caffeine can help you find the energy, it's a good idea to limit this because some of these drinks can have an unhealthy amount of sugars, such as sodas, and aren't directly meant to hydrate you. The baseline to understanding if you're hydrated enough is to look at the color of your urine. If you have a dark yellow color, you're not drinking enough. You want to have a light to lemon yellow color. Hydration is an important part of your workout.

HOW TO FUEL YOUR SYSTEM DURING THE WORKOUT

Unless you're an endurance athlete, you don't need to worry about taking time to eat during your training session. As long as you eat healthy in your pre-workout meal, you won't run into problems during your routine. The best step for you is to focus on staying hydrated because lifting weights can cause you to lose more water than you think. However, if you only plan on training for about a half hour, you shouldn't worry too much about fluids. You might want to stop to get some water a couple of times during your session but it's more important to drink more once you've finished. If you decide to train for over an hour, you will want to include a plan to ensure you get enough liquid nourishment.

You can drink water, but it's more important to ensure you get protein and carbohydrates when you're training for over 60 minutes. Therefore, you want to look at having a sports drink available, specifically about 14 ounces as this contains 25 grams or 7% of your carbohydrate intake. You'll set up certain times to take a drink, such as every half hour. If you feel that you're not performing your best, you're becoming sluggish, or feel too tired to carry on as usual, you will need to increase your liquid intake as these are signs that your glucose is low.

Another diet factor to consider if you're working out for over an hour is calorie intake. It's best to focus on about 50 to 100 calories every half hour to keep your energy up and feeling great. But, you don't want to eat foods that are too heavy for you. The best way to do this is to stick to snacks, such as raisins, low-fat yogurt, or a banana. You can choose to take a quick break, about five to ten minutes, to ensure you get your fuel into your system. It's best to eat and drink slowly because you've been pushing your body and this can create intestinal issues or abdominal pains if you eat too quickly, especially if you need to consume your pre-training meal a few hours prior to the gym.

WHAT TO EAT AFTER WEIGHT TRAINING

You've put a lot of effort into your workout. You probably pushed yourself more than you thought you would or you tried a new weight, making your routine more intense. When this happens, you can cause more tears and damage to your muscles. This makes the need for protein more important, yet you're not sure when you should consume your next meal because there are varying opinions. Some researchers state that you should wait close to three hours while others say you want to consume a protein drink about 30 to 45 minutes later to help muscle repair. Other professionals feel that you need to listen to your body when it comes to your post-workout meal just like you do with your pre-training meal.

One problem is you probably gave more thought to your pre-workout food because you've been told this is the most important meal of your day. While it is important, so is what you consume after you exercise. To give your stomach the least amount of distress and your body the best, you want to understand how you're affected by the workout. The proteins that you consumed prior are now broken down and damaged, especially if you didn't get time to eat your regular meal. Your muscles are partially depleted of the glycogen levels that they're used to because this is what your body uses for fuel during the workout.

Your body will complete its repair and rebuilding process faster if you eat the right nutrients. Eating the right amount of carbs, protein, and even a little fat can help your body restore glycogen, decrease protein breakdown in your muscles, increase muscle growth, and enhance recovery (Semeco, 2016).

So what is the best process to follow when it feels like the professionals can't even agree? Start with the 30 minute window and then pay attention to what your body is telling you. It might be a combination of drinking a sports drink for protein and carbs within the half hour and then eating your meal an hour or two later. You might also find that your stomach and body is strong enough to handle the meal after the 30 minute window. The key is to listen to your body and know what to put in it.

The first step you want to take is to start getting fluids into your system. Without them, you'll become dehydrated and it'll be harder for your body to repair and rebuild itself. You will turn to water right away and then heavier drinks that include protein within the first hour. You want to make sure you drink enough to not only build what you lost but at least 50% more, especially if you regularly exercise. You want to eat at least 100 carbs shortly after you stop exercising. You can do this by consuming about 50 grams within the first 30 minutes and then the rest in the following half hour. When it comes to protein, you want to consume up to 20 grams within the first hour, more if your training was more intense than usual. If you focus on a lighter routine, you can focus more on 10 to 15 grams.

When it comes to foods you can eat, you want to think about your pre-workout meal. If you consumed a heavier meal, such as whole wheat toast and eggs, you might want to look at starting lighter before you go back to the heavy foods. This means you want to stay away from the whole wheat breads and cereals and turn to a little dairy, such as Greek yogurt mixed with seeds or nuts or a banana with a little peanut butter. What this does is help create a balance in your system so you don't have to deal with any abdominal pains. It can also help ensure that you're getting all your food groups in and not focusing on the same foods before and after training. Of course, you also need to consider your weight and how your body handles the foods you're eating. Other options include brown rice, fruit, nut butter, quinoa, chocolate milk, whole grain tortillas, protein powders, and power greens.

TIPS FOR CREATING YOUR MEAL PLAN

Before you get into creating your meal plan, it's important that you do it correctly so you can limit the need to adjust. When beginners start planning their meals around their workout and find that they aren't feeling well, getting dehydrated, or having other issues, they believe that it's not worth it and quickly give up. I want you to succeed in your goals, so let's focus on some of the best advice for planning your meals around weight training.

Timing is everything. One of the first bits of advice a professional will give you is that timing your meals is one of the most important factors. You want to watch what you eat, but when you eat is more important because your foods focus on repairs and building. This means if you only had time for a snack before working out, turn to a full meal within the first half hour after your session ends, if you can. By this point, you might feel that you are starving so it won't be too hard to put fuel into your body.

Don't forget about fats. While healthy fats are more important to eat prior to training, if you don't get them in then you need to include them in your post workout meal. They will help you rebuild your energy as this is its main responsibility in your body. But, you don't want to consume a lot of heart-healthy fats because they contain twice the amount of calories in comparison to protein and carbohydrates.

It's okay to experiment. If you eat the same foods day after day, you will start to struggle with your meal plan. You won't feel like eating the yogurt or drinking the sports drink every single day. It'll be like forcing yourself to eat a certain way causing you to turn away from your diet and weight training. You can keep every factor as fun as possible so you stay motivated. Don't be discouraged when it comes to trying different fruits, nuts, or seeds in your Greek yogurt. It also helps to keep a variety of color in your meals from greens to milky white.

.   .   .

Schedule time for planning and preparing. One of the best ways to continue your meal planning and prepping is to schedule a regular time every week. For instance, if you find that the weekend works best because you can not only go grocery shopping but also come home to prepare, use this time. You might feel that it's best to split it, meaning one day in the week you sit down and create your plan and get a grocery list together. Then you go shopping and prepare by chopping vegetables, cutting chicken, and dividing foods into portions on a different day.

Create a system from the beginning. Sit down and think of the best system for you to use when meal planning. For instance, do you want to establish a journal dedicated to your meal so you know what you liked and didn't like, and how you felt after eating. This can help you know how much you can eat before and after a workout. You might also build an Excel spreadsheet that has your meals so you get the best variety through the month. It can also help you establish what meals your family likes and what they don't really eat. While you might not cut the foods out, you might focus on preparing a different meal for them on a salad night. For instance, if you add chicken to your salad you make them BBQ chicken or chicken with brown rice. This will also give you leftovers for the next day, which makes preparation a bit easier.

EXAMPLE MEAL PLAN

This meal plan will focus on your first week. Each day will have several meals, drinks, and snack ideas. It's not broken down by your pre-working and post-workout meals because the times can be different for you. But, you can easily build in your own meals around your designated exercise time. For example, if you work out after work, you'll want to focus on the snack and dinner whereas in the morning you will focus on breakfast and snack. This meal plan is also just a guide. You can include your favorite foods as long as you count calories, carbs, protein, and fats. You can use it to build a meal plan specialized to your dietary needs, allergies, and any health considerations.

Day 1

Breakfast: One large grapefruit with three eggs, scrambled. You can substitute the grapefruit for a glass of orange juice. Other drinks include coffee, tea, or water.

Snack: Almonds, about 25 to 30 count. This is also the perfect time to ensure you drink a glass of water.

Lunch: Turkey wrap and one apple. Include with a glass of water if you just finished working out within the last half hour or so. A glass of milk is another option.

Snack: Non-fat Greek yogurt and a piece of string cheese with a glass of water or a sports drink.

Dinner: Two cups of snow peas with Thai beef lettuce wraps.

Snack: One Skinny Cow ice cream sandwich—yes! You can still have ice cream!

Day 2

Breakfast: Eggs with a bit of ham and coffee, freshly squeezed juice, or tea.

Snack: 15 baby carrots with hummus or another dip with a glass of water.

Lunch: Two cups of broccoli and Mediterranean hummus wrap with water or a sports drink.

Snack: 1 banana with non-fat Greek yogurt.

Dinner: Tofu stir-fry with one cup of brown rice and

two cups of broccoli. Drink a small glass of milk or
water.

Snack: Apple slices with nut butter.

Day 3

Breakfast: One banana with an omelet scramble with
your favorite morning beverage.

Snack: 10 to 12 cherry tomatoes and a Luna bar with a
glass of water.

Lunch: Leftover tofu stir-fry with one cup of brown
rice with a glass of milk, water, or juice.

Snack: Baby carrots, about 20 to 30.

Dinner: Two cups of broccoli and penne with chicken
Marengo and water.

Snack: Almonds, around 25, with a piece of string
cheese.

Day 4

Breakfast: One grapefruit with French toast. If you
don't like grapefruit you can substitute an orange or
banana. Drink a glass of water or freshly squeezed juice
with a cup of coffee or tea.

Snack: Two boxes of raisins with a glass of water or a
sports drink.

Lunch: Leftover penne with chicken Marengo with one to two cups of broccoli and water.

Snack: Two tablespoons of hummus with 15 baby carrots.

Dinner: Salmon salad with two tablespoons of vinegar dressing or olive oil.

Snack: One Skinny Cow ice cream sandwich.

Day 5

Breakfast: One slice of whole wheat toast with two tablespoons of peanut butter, a banana, and freshly squeezed juice.

Snack: 25 almonds with a glass of water.

Lunch: Turkey wrap and an apple with water or a sports drink.

Snack: One piece of string cheese with a glass of water.

Dinner: Spicy chicken pasta with a side salad. You can pour two tablespoons of vinaigrette or olive oil onto the salad. Have a glass of milk or water to drink.

Snack: One box of raisins.

Day 6

Breakfast: Two to three scrambled eggs with a bowl of fruit and water or freshly squeezed juice.

Snack: One banana and a piece of string cheese with a glass of water.

Lunch: Leftover spicy chicken and pasta with water or milk.

Snack: One cup of broccoli or a protein bar.

Dinner: Veggie burger on a whole wheat bun with a side salad and one serving of sweet potato fries. A glass of water, milk, or even a little wine to drink.

Snack: Non-fat Greek yogurt.

Day 7

Breakfast: Waffles with berries on top and a glass of freshly squeezed juice with water or coffee.

Snack: Carrot sticks with hummus and a glass of water.

Lunch: Salad with 25 almonds.

Snack: 1 Luna Bar with water or a protein shake.

Dinner: Chicken spinach Parmesan with two cups of snow peas, one cup of brown rice, and a glass of water or your favorite drink.

Snack: A piece of string cheese or an apple.

4

OWN THE GYM

Working out at the gym can be intimidating with people who are much further along on their fitness goals. Maybe they have the body you want and you get discouraged. Maybe you don't want to look silly trying to mimic or imitate their workouts. One step you can take to overcome any challenges you face at the gym is to make it simple so your confidence and ability will grow overtime. Always remember that the woman you see with the toned physique and curves in all the right places didn't start working out today. She's been focusing on her routine for years.

One way to help you own the gym is to **keep it simple**. You don't want to start with the exercises that are completed by professionals or people who've been heading to the gym for years. You will reach these routines over time, but it's important to start at a comfortable and easy position and then work yourself to the tougher exercises. After all this is what strength training is all about—building on your skills.

Don't push too far beyond your comfort zone. It's important to push yourself so you continue to grow, but you want to do it a little at a time. You don't need to go from lifting 50 pounds to 150 pounds in a year. You always need to keep your comfort zone in your line of vision or you can find yourself giving up and walking away. Comfort is an important feeling when it comes to completing tasks that make you feel nervous. You can also find yourself thinking negatively when it comes to working out, which is an emotion you always want to avoid.

Focus on proper form and not weights. When you walk into the gym, you're probably more concerned with how much you can lift, but this isn't where your mind should be at this point. You need to focus on form. It's more important to get comfortable on how to handle the machines and keeping your form proper. Once you have a strong form, you can then move on to building your muscles.

TIPS TO OVERCOME FEELING JUDGED AT THE GYM

If you fear the gym because you're afraid of judgment, you're not alone. A recent survey by Fitrated shows that about 65% of women don't go to the gym because of this feeling (Lexington

Healing Arts Academy, 2019). If you do go to the gym, you might hide in a corner and constantly watch other people. You see someone coming toward you and your anxiety spikes as you wonder if they're walking by or they want to critique your form or exercise routine. You probably stop working out, give a fake smile, and a sigh of relief as they continue walking. If you notice someone looking in your direction, you stop working out, check your phone, take a drink of water, or don't put as much effort into your routine. When someone else starts using equipment next to you, it's time to move to another area where people aren't around you. Fortunately, you don't need to hold onto this feeling because there are many ways to start taking control of this feeling.

Don't go to the gym alone. If you have a friend that wants to start working out and you can go together, do it. Even if you both worry about what other people will think, you're not alone and this can ease your anxiety. You might also find a workout buddy in the gym, maybe someone else you see sitting on the sidelines when you look in their direction.

Search for the best gym. If you live in a small city, you might not have an option for a gym. However, it never hurts to look outside of your neighborhood. It's always possible that the place that makes you feel more secure is about 15 to 20 minutes away. While this isn't always ideal when you have one within walking distance from your work or home, it is important to find a gym that makes you feel comfortable. For example, maybe the gym further away has a higher rate of bodybuilders that are willing and able to help you. They might also have classes that fit your needs.

Get a tour of the gym before you settle on a membership. Contact the gyms you are looking at and ask them if you can schedule a tour and to talk with the owner or a personal trainer. They can help make you comfortable. Chances are high they'll know people at the gym and introduce you, which can make your first time working out feel less intimidating. They might also agree to help you with form and getting started as a member. If it's possible, ask them to show you how the machines work so you have a good idea when it comes to form and you feel more confident using the equipment from day one.

Use the breathing strategy. It will take time to overcome your fear. Unfortunately, it's not something that will happen overnight or by taking a tour of the gym. While a tour can help, many women continue to struggle with anxiety or "fitness fear" for a period of time—even when they have confidence in their form and know how to use the equipment. It doesn't always happen often, but sometimes you'll be in the gym and it'll feel crowded or you'll feel the worry happen when you're trying a new routine. In these moments, you want to find a quiet corner and focus on your breathing. Close your eyes and take a few deep breaths before you get back to your routine.

Look for success stories. When you're walking around with the personal trainer learning about the gym and equipment, ask them about any personal stories of success. They might know a few people who would be willing to talk to you or share their personal story. When you hear about someone else who walked a similar journey to yours, you'll start to feel more confident that you can accomplish your goals.

Women's fitness groups. You can probably find some general women's fitness groups on social media and they're a great advantage for you. You'll meet people in the group who can help you gain confidence and troubleshoot when you're not sure where to turn in your routine. They can also help you stay motivated and give you advice. However, it's also important to join local groups as they can exercise with you, making you less likely to feel alone at the gym.

Keep your eyes on your goals. One of the best ways to stay focused and motivated is to remember why you joined the gym. You can do this by writing your fitness goals down or even creating a vision board so you can visually see your goal every day. For example, you might put your ideal weight on the board along with pictures of equipment or trainers. You can even put words on it, such as "be stronger," "be healthier," "look better," and "feel better."

Think Positively. I realize this is easier said than done, but the more you focus on positivity around you, the stronger your confidence will become in the gym. This means that you want to keep people in your life who want you to succeed. They are your cheerleaders when you're struggling to head to the gym, maybe by coming with you or just telling you that you're doing an excellent job and to keep going. It also means that you want to focus on positive thoughts, even when you don't get your form correct the first time or you thought you were ready to try a new exercise but you're not. For example, instead of saying, "I can't do this" you'll tell yourself, "I couldn't do it today, but with hard work and dedication, I will accomplish it later."

Don't compare. Social comparisons are a problem for a lot of people. You've probably caught yourself looking at a personal trainer or someone at the gym, or even at the grocery store, and thought "If only I had her confidence" or "If only I could look like her." It's important to remember that everyone looks and is built differently. For instance, you might have a bigger bone structure than someone else. You might have a health condition that causes you to gain weight easily and makes it harder to keep off. Instead of focusing on someone else, you need to focus on the most important person in your life—you.

WHAT EXERCISES ARE BEST FOR ME AT THE GYM?

It's intimidating to walk into a gym and see rows of exercise equipment. You can have motivation to start your workout routine but find yourself anxious the minute you step through the doors. Take a deep breath and realize there is no need to change your mind because help is available to you in many forms. Not only can you talk to a professional trainer but most of the equipment at the gym will have an explanation of what muscles are targeted and how to use them.

Free weights and machines are the two categories of weight training in the gym. There are several studies that prove both will help you increase muscle mass. In July 2019 *Experimental Gerontology* published an article that revealed you can build strength with any type of weight lifting machine (Halse, 2020). There isn't one that will help you build faster, but there are differences when it comes to a beginner. In fact, it's best for you to start with machines because they're designed to help you through your training. One seeming problem you may run into is your height as the machines are not designed for women of average height, however the majority of the machines are adjustable.

Free weights include barbells, medicine balls, dumbbells, and kettlebells. You don't need to be a certain height to fit with them comfortably and they don't constrain your movements. Understanding the correct form is more essential because free weights require more effort on your part. It is harder to learn from free weights because you need to have more control over your body but they can also teach you more about how to employ functional movements correctly.

The biggest factor to remember when lifting weights is that the key to avoiding injury and faster gains is proper form. It's challenging to notice your form unless you're looking into a mirror during your exercise, which still allows you to miss some of the function because you can only change what you see. Plus, there is always a possibility that you're not performing the exercise correctly when you think you are (simple and common beginner's mistake). For your best safety and education in the weight room, it's best you have a personal trainer or workout buddy who has more experience to help guide you.

HOW TO GET STARTED IN THE GYM

Now is the time to start putting your dreams into motion by designing a weight training program. When you're first starting, you want to look toward total-body workouts so you can get all your muscles moving. You'll also learn the best form for your whole body, which will help you when it comes to the details of a work out for each area. It also lets you ease into a weekly workout routine because you can limit your gym sessions to two to three.

Step one: Determine your overall fitness goal. What is the main reason you want to get in shape? Is it to lose weight or for your health? This goal might change over time, so it's okay to focus on your goal for the next month or so. Think about what changes you want to see within the next few weeks. Be sure to include your diet plan! You don't need to write out your full meal plan, but keep in mind how your diet will help your fitness and health goals.

Step two: Create SMART goals. You can make your overall goal into reasonable steps following the **S**pecific, **M**easurable, **A**ttainable, **R**ealistic, **T**imely technique. You want to be detailed in this step. For example, instead of saying you want to lose weight, you'll say, "I want to lose 4% of my body fat in two months." The key is to ensure that you can reach this goal within the timeframe. You'll then discuss how you will go about this, such as weighing yourself weekly, going to the gym so many days a week, walking in the morning, etc. Don't worry about having to include certain exercises in this moment.

Step three: How many days will you dedicate to the weight room? Analyze your goals and think about how often you'll need to lift weights, but be realistic. If you have days where you can't really get away from other responsibilities, don't commit to going to the gym right now. You can always add it in down the road if time opens up or you adjust your schedule. But, you don't want to come up with excuses either. You need to ensure you set aside time a few days out of the week. For example, you might write down five days because you have time before work every morning. You might choose three as a starting point and increase your days once you get more comfortable and focused on training. Write it down in your daily planner or phone, and set alarms to help you follow through.

Step four: Think about the cardio. Your goals might not focus heavily on cardio, but this doesn't mean you should ignore it. Maybe you'll choose to walk during the days you don't make it to the gym. You might even include these exercises in your home. For example, you'll dedicate 30 minutes three days a week to yoga, walking, or cycling. You can also include a few minutes of cardio to help get your blood moving when you walk into the gym.

Step five: Choose your exercises for the first few weeks. You'll learn more about the exercises in the next few chapters, but it's important to leave a space in your plan so you can write down the ones you want to focus on. You're not going to choose exercises that you'll do for months or a year. As a beginner, you'll focus on the first month or two. You can choose as many exercises as you think you can handle and that's safe for your body (remember it's okay to adjust later). But, you can also start with six to eight different exercises to ensure you're working your upper and lower body.

Step six: Repeat for several weeks. Finally, set a deadline for this plan, such as two months. At this point, you'll follow the plan and when your deadline comes, you'll evaluate where you are and adjust to fit your new needs.

PROPER FORM IS KEY

No matter what type of weight lifting you're focusing on, whether machines or free weights, you always need to use proper form because it's the key to better gains and keeping your body injury free. But, you also need to understand your individual differences, such as your body type, mobility, limb length, flexibility, and injury history. For example, if you've broken your ankle previously, you might have trouble with it during some exercises. Maybe you can't move it well on one side or you start to get pain, which means you're not following your proper form. Another example is squats. Some people believe a squat is when your thighs and hips are parallel to the floor, while others go down further. Both of these are correct; it all depends on your flexibility. You're an individual, which means your proper form is different from your workout buddy's. There is no universal form that is perfect for everyone, but this doesn't make understanding this process harder. In fact, it's easier because you learn what feels to you and your body will guide you.

One of the main reasons proper form fails is because it's not discussed during training. Professional trainers will always talk about your form during your first session and help you understand how to get there. They will guide you as long as you include them in your workout time. But, when you start training without help or knowledge of what's best for you, you're less likely to follow through with the right form. You can also find yourself injured early in the process, which can lead you to deciding that strength training is not right for you. It's best to train with someone who has more experience but also remember to ask someone if you are not sure your form is correct.

Another reason it fails is sacrificing your form to progress quickly. Taking time to ensure you're lifting correctly for your body type can take a bit of adjustment, so you don't start your intense workout right away. This can be frustrating because you feel it will take you longer to get the results you want, but it's essential to go the slower route. In the long run, you'll feel and see better results when you follow proper form over quick progress.

Proper form is important for two main reasons:

1. It decreases injuries, which goes beyond pulling a muscle. You can also hurt yourself by performing too many exercises in one session or not allowing your body to recover. Pushing yourself to complete a routine isn't the best for your body because of a previous injury or joint trouble. For example, if you have a lot of shoulder pain you want to be cautious of exercises focusing on this area so you don't cause further injury. You can also have an accident, such as dropping a weight on your foot or using too much weight on the bench press without a spotter. You

should always have a spotter for safety reasons because it's possible that you can get stuck and then you can't lift the weights off of yourself. If you're alone and want to bench press, don't push yourself by adding weight, stick with what you know you can safely handle or ask someone nearby in the gym to watch out for you. It's always better to be safe than sorry! The most common reason for injuries is bad form. For instance, if you're not mindful about your form and what you're doing or you learned from a bad source, such as a YouTube video where the trainer wasn't a professional (not all videos are good), you added too much weight, or you're tired. Near the end of your training your body and mind are fatigued, which causes you to pay less attention to your form, or you're just not putting the same amount of effort into it.

2. You train the right group of muscles in connection to your goals. If you're lifting weights to improve your curves, you don't want to just focus on how much you can lift; you need to focus on effectively training your muscles. Many people overlook this point because they think the more weight they can lift the better their body will look. No, if you don't use proper form, you won't get your desired results. This is why it's important to make your goals and intentions clear in your plan and to any trainer. How can you tell if you're not using the right muscles effectively? The way they

feel. For example, if you want to focus on your back so you incorporate pull-ups and lat pull downs but you feel your biceps more than your back muscles, your form isn't proper. You need to feel the muscles you're working on. They have to get the workout.

Where can you go to learn proper form?

Find a personal trainer. You want to find someone who is listening to your goals and understands that each weight lifter's form is different. Finding someone who knows what they're doing can take a bit of time, especially when it comes to scheduling sessions. For example, if you work every day from eight to five, you need to find someone willing to meet you around your work day and maybe during the weekend. Not every trainer will follow your day as they might have set hours they work at the gym. You might go through a couple of trainers before you find the right one for you. You'll know they're your trainer because you'll feel comfortable with them and they'll take time to show you how to exercise. They will also have credentials. It's hard to know who the best trainer is when you're getting started, but if you notice that you're not feeling the right muscles working or any other signs that you're not their priority during the session, keep looking.

Have your form evaluated by a professional. You don't need to spend the money on a trainer if you can't afford to, but you can request they take time to evaluate your form. Once you have learned everything you need to from this book, you'll start training and this is when you request an evaluation. You can ask a trainer to come to one of your sessions or find someone who will watch a video of you perform.

Teach yourself from watching videos. The problem with videos is you can find a lot of bad ones that seem good. Take your time when it comes to searching for videos so you know you can find ones that are the best for you. Another way to start is by finding websites to some of the most notable trainers, such as Jillian Michaels. You should still look for someone to double-check your form. In a sense, you're teaching yourself through videos and this can lead you to understanding a part incorrectly or missing something important. The best way to teach yourself is to watch what you're doing, so you want to have a mirror and notice all of your angles, not just one. You also need to know what mistakes you can make and be aware of them—be knowledgeable about strength training. Know how you can correct the mistakes you make or who to contact for help. You also need to be willing to accept any mistakes. It's not always easy to notice what you do wrong or admit it. Don't tell yourself, "It's okay, I'll fix it eventually." You want to fix your form immediately.

5

SCULPTING A TONED UPPER BODY
WITHOUT BULKING UP

Before you start with any exercises, it's important that you know you don't need to worry about getting too bulky. A woman's hormones and anatomy aren't genetically designed to put on large amounts of muscle due to lack of testosterone. You can lift weights every day for your designated time frame and feel your mindset change as you begin to gain the physique that you want.

One of the best features about lifting is you can randomize your workout routine or you can primarily look at the areas you want to build curves. You can focus on your back every day, but build in different workouts throughout the week. For example, you might do the reverse fly on Monday and Thursday; the single-leg deadlift with row on Tuesday and Friday; plank with row on Wednesday and Saturday; and choosing your favorite exercise for Sunday (or just taking a break because that's important too). Of course, you can always decide to focus on your arms on Monday, shoulders Tuesday, back on Wednesday, etc.

BACK

Before you step into back training, you need to understand the problems that can arise so you can take the best care of yourself. First, it's easy to find yourself stuck in the same routine because you feel overwhelmed by the volume of variations, but you want to mix it up. You need to work all of your back muscles along with the rest of your upper and lower body. To help yourself overcome this challenge, know what you want to achieve before you start lifting or have a general idea. For example, if you don't want to tone your back too much at the start, what area do you want to work on? If it's your arms, focus more on arm exercises in your routine and include back a couple days out of your week. In a few months you might be more interested in working on your back muscles, so you incorporate them more.

The second problem is that women tend to start exercising without giving a thought to what muscles they are building. It's important that you understand your anatomy and get to know your back muscles.

Other muscles in the back include:

- *Latissimus dorsi* is the largest muscle in the back and can dictate your overall physique. You can separate the large muscle into two smaller areas, known as the low and high lats. The low lats show strength and thickness. They connect on your lower back whereas high lats focus on your upper back, giving it its width.

- *Teres minor and infraspinatus* are two smaller muscles that are part of your rotator cuff. They help rotate and extend the shoulder. If you're having trouble with your shoulders or you have a career where you overwork them, you want to perform exercises focused on these muscles regularly to help ease any tension and overuse.

- *Teres major* is located in the upper back and often referred to as a bubbly muscle. Its main job is to assist the lats.

- *Posterior deltoid* works closely with your shoulders during extension. For example, when you stretch your arm behind your body, you're focusing on these muscles.

- *Lower, upper, and mid trapezius* muscles retract, elevate, and depress the shoulder bone or scapula. It's important to be aware of your form because you can spend more time working your upper trapezius over the others, which can lead to strained or damaged muscles over time.

- *Major and minor rhomboids* also focus on the shoulder blades. Take a moment to squeeze your shoulder blades together. These are the muscles you feel working to create scapular retraction and scapular downward rotation.

Another way to look at these muscles is to sort them into three categories:

1. *Flexor muscles* attach to the front of the spine. They are part of your abdominal muscles and allow you to arch and lift your lower back. They also help you bend forward or flex, like when you're showing off your muscles. If you want to increase the curvature of your lower back and get the bonus of tightening your abs, you'll focus on these muscles during your workout.
2. *Extensor muscles* attach to the back of the spine. When you lift objects or stand you're using these muscles.
3. *Oblique muscles* attach to the side of the spine and help it rotate.

To give your back the best workout and ensure you're working all of your muscles you want to focus on various exercises throughout your routine, but you can also favor specific areas to get the curves you want. For instance, if you want to broaden your shoulder blades, then you'll look at managing your rhomboid and trapezius muscles. If you want to focus on making your torso look and feel narrower, you'll spend more time on high lats.

Lat Pull-Down

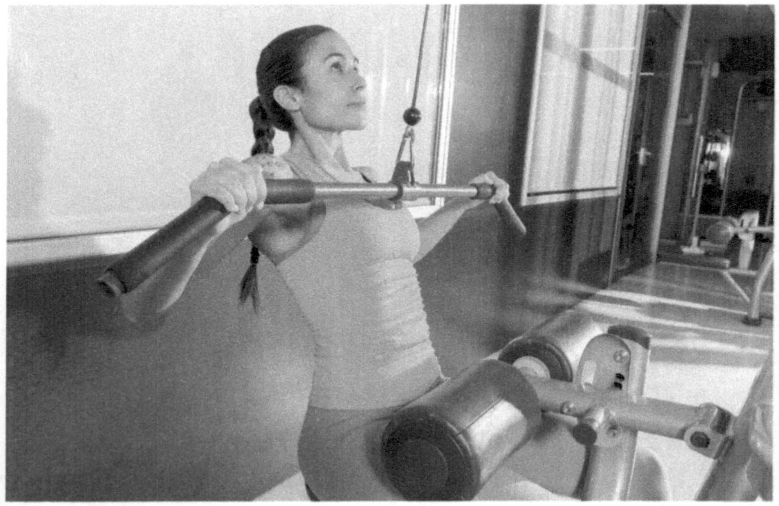

The lat pull-down is performed on a machine and focuses on the latissimus dorsi muscles. It's one of the easiest exercises to learn and will help you build strength in your back. You do need to grip so if you have trouble with your hands you can wear wrist straps. Normally people do about a dozen reps per set.

1. Sit down at a pull-bar machine that has a wide bar attached to a pulley.

2. Take time to adjust the knee pad of the machine to your size as they will keep you from being pulled up. They will also help you stay in proper form.

3. With your palms facing forward, grab the bar at the best grip zone for you. For example, if you want a medium grip you need to have your hands spaced so they're parallel to your shoulders. A wider grip has your hands spaced wider than your shoulders, whereas a close grip is smaller than your shoulder width.

4. Once your hands are in place, bring your shoulders back about 30 degrees so you have a curve with your lower back. Your chest should be sticking out. Keep this as your starting position.

5. When you exhale, pull the bar down to your upper chest. Keep the upper arms down and back while drawing at your shoulders. To help with your posture, notice the feeling you have in your back muscles. You should feel like you're squeezing them. Don't move your upper torso as the only part of you that should be mobile are your arms. Your forearms need to hold the bar, which is their only job so don't pull down with your forearms.

6. Once you feel the muscles between your shoulders squeezing, inhale, and then gradually bring your arms back to the starting position.

7. Repeat for the rest of your reps.

Bent-Over Dumbbell Rear Delt Row

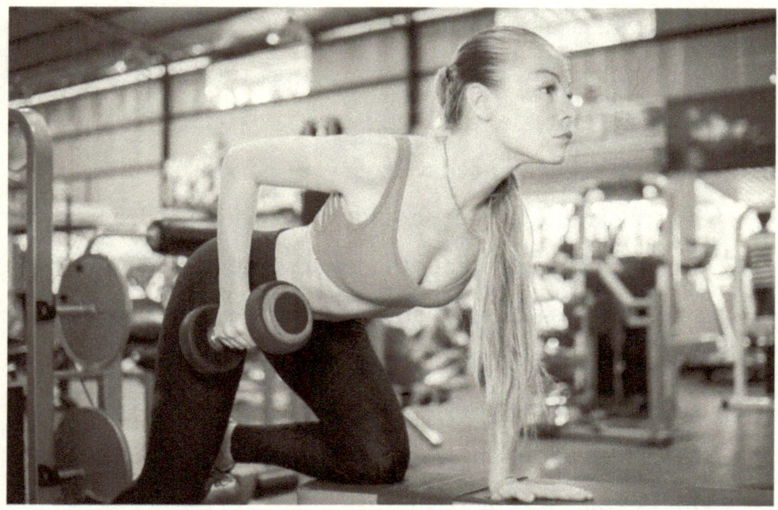

This exercise focuses on the back of the shoulder joint, especially the rear and medial heads of the deltoid. You'll start with this movement if you want to balance out the development of your shoulders. You should aim to perform at least 15 reps during each set.

1. Start by standing straight with a dumbbell in each hand.

2. Bend your knees slightly, allowing your body to flex at the hip so you can lean forward. But, you need to keep your back straight throughout the exercise routine.

3. Your arms should hang perpendicular with the floor. Point your elbows at your sides and pronate your

wrist, similar to a palm facing the back of you. This is your starting position.

4. Your movement will be extending your shoulder, flexing your elbows, and rowing the dumbbells to shoulder height.

5. Make sure you squeeze your scapulae together while moving and keep your shoulders retracted.

6. Your upper arms need to be perpendicular to your torso.

7. Keep rowing until your elbows are inside of 90 degrees and pause.

8. Slowly bring your arms back to their starting position, but don't stand up until you are done with your reps.

The Pull-Up

The pull-up strengthens the muscles of your biceps, core, grip, lats, and upper back. You don't need to have an exercise machine, but you do need to have a bar or something to grab onto. It's possible to exercise at different grip variations, as long as you're comfortable and not causing injury. It's important to note that many women can't do one pull-up when they start working out and that's okay because it creates a goal that you can work up to.

1. Grab the pull-up handles or bar with an overhand grip.

2. Keep your hands so they're more than shoulder width apart. You're now at your starting position.

3. Lift yourself up by flexing your elbows and retracting your shoulder blades. Pull your chest up but keep your back straight the whole time. It also helps to keep your head neutral.

4. If needed, tuck your legs under you to help your grip with the bar without moving the rest of your body.

5. Lower your body back to your starting position.

6. Repeat for as many reps as you choose.

Cable Seated Rows

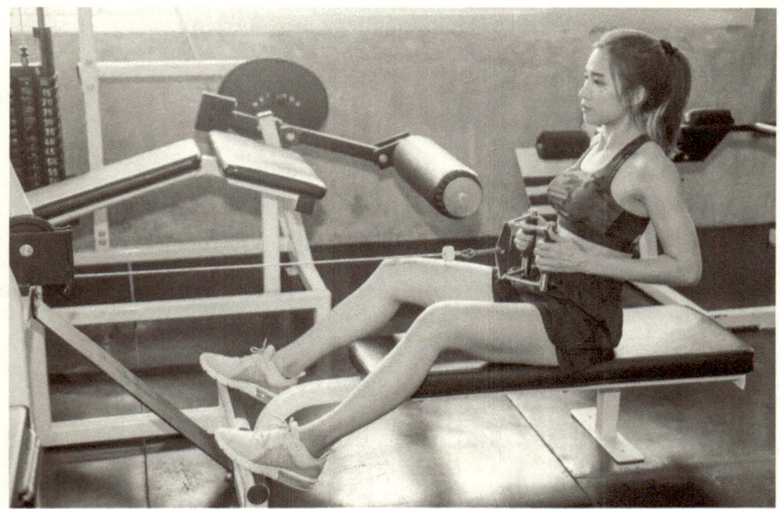

The seated cable row will help you work out your middle and upper back. It can also target your biceps, but to a lesser degree. It's one of the most popular muscle-building routines so you can easily find the necessary equipment (and someone to help you if needed) in any gym. Like the other exercises where you grip, you can use a variety of lengths to find the most comfortable place for yourself.

1. Sit down on the bench and face a cable pulley.
2. Place your feet firmly on the floor or footrest but ensure that your knees are slightly bent.
3. Grab one of the handles in each hand and make sure your palms are facing inward. Keep your back straight throughout the routine. This is your starting position.
4. Pull the cable by moving your elbows back, but close to your body. Pull until your elbows are a bit beyond your side and hold for a couple of seconds.
5. Exhale and let the pulley move back, bringing yourself back to your starting position.
6. Repeat this process until you've completed your reps.

SHOULDERS

There are several important points on the shoulder that you'll use during exercise to help you strengthen and balance this part of your body. One is the shoulder joint, which consists of several muscles and bones, such as the scapula (shoulder blade behind you), humerus (bone of the upper arm), and collarbone. The shoulder joint is around the humerus and fits into an indent in the scapula. There are several muscles around the bones. One of the most common injuries is on the shoulder because of all the little muscles and bones included. As long as you use correct form and allow your muscles to heal after an intense workout, you'll limit any chances of injury. The rotator cuff is another important location and includes four muscles known as the infraspinatus. It will work with the rest of the shoulder to keep everything stable.

Don't forget about your shoulder muscles. "The delts" or deltoid is a common term that refers to the triangular muscle group covering the shoulder joint. It stretches from the top of your shoulder to the clavicle and then down the scapula and then attached to the bone of the upper arm (Body Building, 2018). There are smaller portions of the deltoid:

- **Anterior** rotates the arm toward the middle of the body. It will also lift the arm in the front. You'll work this muscle when you face your palms down and in.
- **Lateral** is used when you're lifting your arm away from your body, such as raising it from your side and out, as if you were trying to hold on to something. It's usually strengthened when you're using a wide grip during exercises.
- **Rear** is a focus when you're moving your arm in an outward motion or behind your body.

Side Lateral Raise

You'll use dumbbells for this exercise to help you balance out your shoulders while building muscle and strength. It doesn't matter what size weights you use because even the lightest will help make this part of your body appear more developed and wider. Another benefit is that you can perform this workout while standing or sitting down. The main focus is your medial head of the deltoid.

1. Stand straight and hold a dumbbell in each hand. Keep the weights at the side with the palms of your hands in your direction. This is your starting position.
2. Lift the dumbbells up by keeping your arms and back straight. The only part of your body you should use to move your arms are your shoulders.
3. When you lift, exhale and raise your arms up until they're equal to your shoulders. Ensure your palms are down when you're lifting.
4. Inhale and gradually lower your arms back down to the starting point. Remember to keep your neck neutral.
5. Repeat this motion until you've completed the reps.

Alternating Dumbbell Front Raise

The main benefit is it develops your anterior deltoids. It also lets you get more reps within each set because you'll rest one arm while the other one is working. Usually you'll perform at least a dozen repetitions within each set, but you can always do more. The challenge is understanding when to stop so you don't overwork certain muscles or cause an injury.

1. Pick up a couple of dumbbells and hold one in each hand. Keep your body straight and allow your arms to rest with your elbows pointed away from your body. You should hold the weights so the palms of your hands are facing you and let the weights rest on your thighs. This is your starting position.
2. Raise one dumbbell in front while keeping your arm extended and your back straight until it's at shoulder height. Keep your palms facing down.
3. Slowly lower your arm without bending it, moving your back, or your head. Then lift the weight in the opposite arm in the same manner.
4. Repeat this process until you are done with your repetitions.

Seated Dumbbell Press

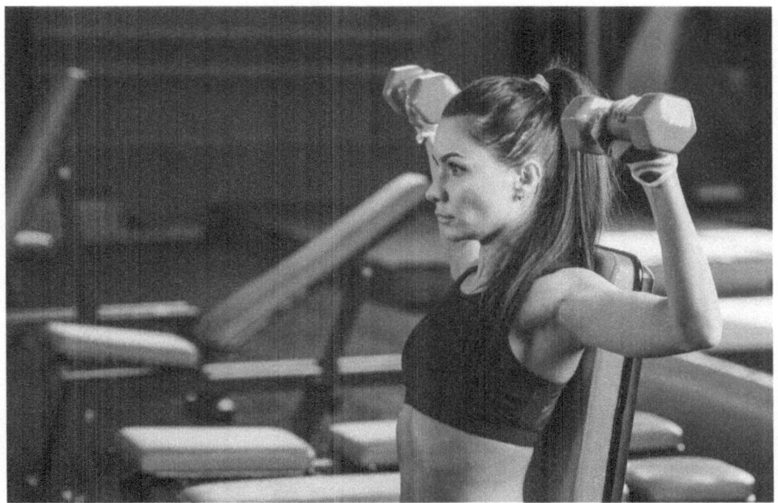

While most of this exercise builds your front heads, your triceps will also feel some burn. This is sometimes used with barbells, but many trainers feel that you can reduce the chances of hurting yourself by using dumbbells, especially when you're still learning your proper form.

1. Sit down on a bench with or without back support. When you're beginning, the support can help you keep your back straight. Pick up a dumbbell and place one in each hand.
2. Lift the dumbbells up to your shoulders by rotating your arms out so your wrists are facing outward. This is your starting position.

3. As you begin to lift the weights over your head, exhale while keeping your neck neutral and your back straight. Lift them until your arms are extended up. If you're having trouble holding the weights, try it with lighter dumbbells.

4. Lower your control by slowly bringing your arms back down, bending at your elbows until you reach the starting position.

5. Repeat this process until you've done all your repetitions.

Machine Rear Delt Fly

You can add strength to your head of the deltoids. It will also help build the muscles in your upper back. Start with smaller weights because this exercise is meant to focus on the smaller muscles in your shoulders. You can use the machine chest fly to perform this exercise, but you'll need to sit facing the opposite direction. It's best to aim to do at least 15 repetitions, but you can always add more. Using this technique, you'll build balanced, healthy-looking shoulders.

1. Make sure that the handles are fully to the back of the machine and sit down so you are facing the handles. Grab the handle bars with your hands facing forward and palms facing down. Keep your feet firmly on the floor and your shoulders level with the handles. You're now at your starting position.

2. Exhale and push the handles to the sides and then behind you. Keep the palms facing down and your arms extended. Rotate the machine with your shoulders and not your elbows. Your back should be straight at all times and your legs should not move.

3. Inhale and bring your arms back so they are centered in front of you in the starting position.

4. Repeat this process as many times as you set.

Smith Machine Shoulder Press

This is another shoulder exercise with machines that targets the deltoid muscles. You should complete at least a dozen reps in one setting to add size and strength to your shoulders. If you worry about dropping the bar on your chest, this is a great place to start because it's said to help you gain strength while making you comfortable so you stop worrying. It's also easier to move the bar and keep your position because it moves on track.

1. Start by sitting on a bench, use one with back support to help your form. Move the bar's height so it's equal with your chest.

2. Face your palms forward with your wrists stacked over your elbows, so you can easily pick up the bar. Keep your feet flat on the floor.

3. Exhale and lift the barbell, pushing up with your upper arms and shoulders to give your muscles the best

strength. Raise it until your arms are fully extended. You are now at the starting position.

4. While keeping your neck neutral and your back straight, inhale and then lower the bar until it's even with your chin.

5. Repeat for the recommended number of repetitions.

ARMS

Your biceps are a part of the upper arm that gets a lot of movement, especially when you're pulling. It includes the brachialis and brachioradialis. One of their main functions is to flex the elbow and the other is to move your wrist closer to your face. They connect to various points in the shoulder, so you can help build some of these muscles while focusing on arm exercises. There are two main muscles in your biceps: long and short head. You'll focus on the long head when your exercises have your arms at the side. When your arms are in front of you, you'll improve your short head muscle, which is under the long head and directly under your armpit.

When you push and extend, you're working your triceps. They have three heads—lateral, deep or medial, and long. The long head is located on the right side of your upper arm.

EZ-Bar Skullcrusher

Don't worry, the bar won't actually crush your skull! The bar will come down toward your forehead while building your tricep muscles. If you have trouble with your wrists, this is a great exercise to focus on and it's perfect when you need to focus on lighter weights.

1. Lay flat on a bench with an EZ bar straight up over your shoulders. Some people use a straight bar, but this can be worse on your wrists. Hold the bar so your palms are facing up toward the ceiling as this will give you the best grip.
2. Keep your back straight with your feet flat on the floor. You're now in your starting position.
3. Inhale and lower the bar by hinging your elbows toward your forehead while keeping your shoulders lined up with your elbows that are stationary.
4. When you start to straighten your elbows to bring the bar back to starting position, exhale.
5. Repeat for as many reps as you're recommended to do.

Cable Overhead Triceps Extension

This is another exercise that aims to strengthen and build your triceps. You can use light to moderate weight as the cable gives your muscles consistent tension to help them workout. Along with all three of the tricep muscles, the long head will receive the most attention. You should do at least eight to twelve reps in a set.

1. If the rope isn't attached to the bottom of the pulley machine, attach it.

2. Using both hands, grab the rope and raise your hands directly above your head. You should be standing with your back toward the machine. Your palms should be facing each other and knuckles aimed at the ceiling.

3. Make sure that your elbows are extended and close to your head. You want your arms perpendicular to the floor. You're now at the starting position.

4. Inhale and gradually lower the rope so it starts to go behind your head, bend your elbows with the cable while keeping your upper arms in the same position. Don't move your back or your head; just bend your elbows.

5. Bring your arms back to the starting position as you exhale. Notice how your triceps feel when you're performing this exercise.

6. Repeat for the number of repetitions recommended.

Cross Body Hammer Curl

This will not only build your biceps but also both the brachialis and brachioradialis. Your forearm will thicken as it focuses on the long head. You strengthen these muscles because you'll lift the weights across your torso and not directly in front of your body. The key is to keep your wrist neutral just like you do when you're hammering a nail into the wall. You should complete between ten to twelve reps per set.

1. Sit straight while holding a dumbbell in each hand. You want your palms facing in with your arms down at your sides. This is your starting position.

2. With your palms continuing to face in, exhale and begin to lift your lower right arm without twisting it. Curl the weight toward your left shoulder while keeping your back straight. Make sure that your upper arm, between your shoulder and elbow remains stationary. Hold the position for a second.

3. Inhale and gradually lower the weight back to the starting position.

4. Repeat the same movement but with your left arm and aiming toward your right shoulder.

5. Continue this alternating process as you complete the number of reps you choose.

Standing Dumbbell Triceps Extension

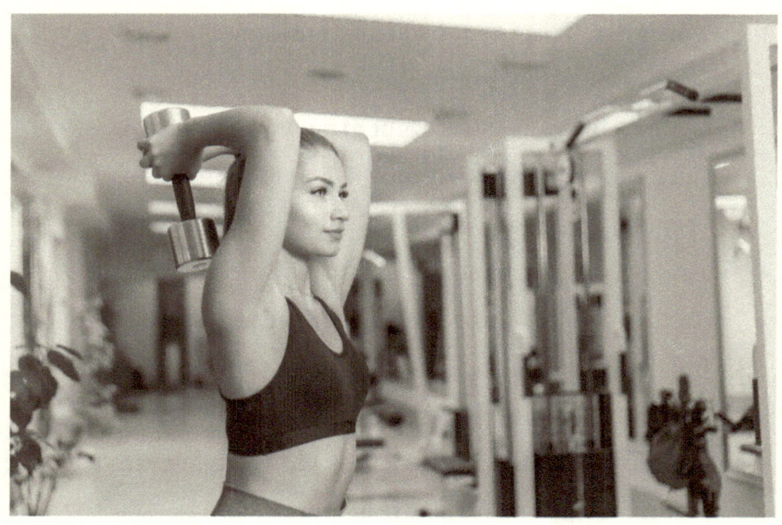

This exercise is done with one dumbbell at any amount of weight. You'll focus on all three of the muscles within your triceps and even help your shoulders gain a little strength, but not as much as your arms. You should do between eight to twelve repetitions in one set.

1. Stand up with a dumbbell of a light to moderate weight in your hand. Spread your legs a bit while you straighten up your back and set your neck in a neutral position.

2. Lift your arms all the way up while holding one end of the dumbbell between your hands. Your hands should be above your head but the weight behind you. Have

your palms facing the ceiling so the weight is resting in them. Close your fingers tight enough so you don't drop the weight behind you. This is your starting position.

3. Exhale and slowly lower the dumbbell down, behind your back. Keep your shoulders and elbows stationary and don't arch your back. The only movement should be your lower arms.

4. Once the free end of the weight is between your shoulder blades, raise the weight back up to the starting position.

5. Repeat this process until you're done with the set.

Triceps Pushdown

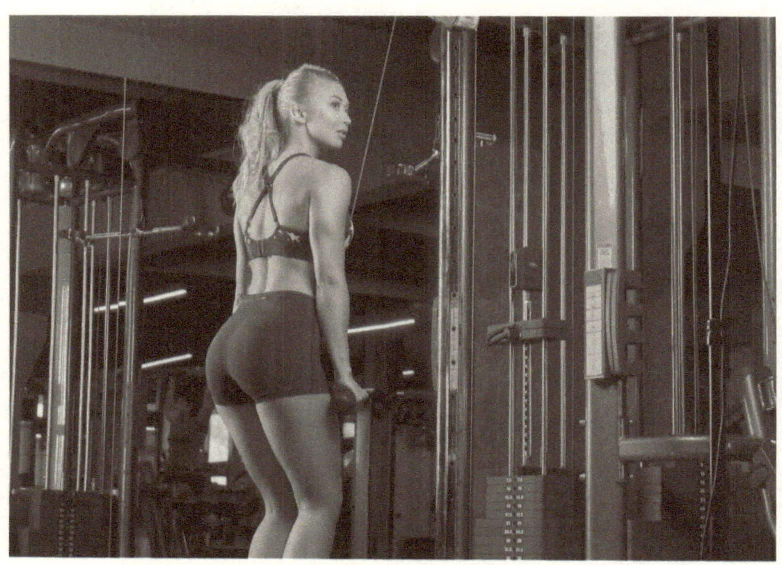

You use a machine with a cable v-bar. This exercise lets you add on more weight than what you usually use, but you still need to be cautious and considerate of your muscles and body. You will work all of your tricep muscles, but the lateral head receives the moves work. The number of repetitions you should focus on in each set is between eight to twelve.

1. Attach an angled or straight bar to a high pulley.
2. Grab the bar with your palms facing down in an overhand manner. You want to keep the length shoulder width.
3. Keep your torso straight with your legs and feet separated a little. Pull your arms to your side and bend your elbows to 90 degrees. This is your starting position.
4. Exhale while you push the bar down by extending your elbows. Bring the bar down so it touches your thighs. Keep your arms perpendicular to the floor and make sure your elbows, shoulders, and back remain stationary.
5. Hold the contracted position for a second before you start slowly bringing the bar back up to the starting position.
6. Repeat until you're done with the set.

ABS/CORE

Training your abs is probably high on your list but they can also be the exercises you struggle with most because, well, even experienced trainers struggle with them. It's not everyone's favorite type of exercises, but you'll start to feel the results quickly, especially when it comes to the soreness of your muscles.

The rectus abdominis is one of the core muscles. It's most commonly called the "six pack" and includes both the upper and lower abs. It is responsible for twisting your torso down and forward along with pulling up your knees toward your torso.

The muscles that run down the sides of your body between your lats and rectus abdominis are called the obliques. They not only focus on contracting and extending your torso laterally, but also twist you from side to side.

Above the obliques and beside your rib cage are the intercostals. They work closely with the rib cage to expand and contract it.

If you continue moving up and a bit to the side of the rib cage, you can feel small muscles that will remind you of three fingers. They run from the side of the rib cage to the lats and are called the serratus. Their job is to help your shoulder move forward as much as possible (Perine, 2020).

Kneeling Cable Crunch

This is another exercise that will focus on your upper abs. You can start with less weight and still feel the benefits. Of course, you'll want to gradually add weight so you continue to strengthen your abs. It's similar to the traditional crunch. You should do about eight to twelve repetitions in one set.

1. Make sure that the pulley has a rope attachment.
2. Kneel below the pulley, facing away from the machine.
3. Hold the ends of the rope attachment over your shoulders. You're now at the starting position.
4. Exhale and bend at the waist so you can contract your abs while leaning your elbows toward your thighs. Keep your form as straight as possible while in motion so you don't bend your back.
5. Ensure you pull the rope down when you crunch and keep your hips up with your neck in a neutral position.
6. Inhale and bring yourself back to the starting point.
7. Repeat for as many times as you need for your set.

Hanging Leg Raise

With this exercise you will focus on the lower abs. One of the benefits is that you can perform it anywhere there is a bar that you can safely hang from. Not only will it help your lower abs, but you can also work your leg and arm muscles as well, just not as strongly. You should do about a dozen repetitions in one set.

1. Extend your arms up to grab a bar so you can hang there. Make sure it's tall enough so your feet are hanging off of the floor. If you're grabbing two handles, ensure that your palms are facing each other. This is your starting position.

2. Exhale and bend your knees to lift your legs so you can contract your abs. Bring your knees up toward your core area while keeping your back straight and your neck neutral.

3. Inhale and lower your legs back to the starting position.

4. Repeat for as many repetitions as recommended.

Seated Bar Twist

This exercise is used to strengthen the obliques. It will help you build core resiliency and strength. It can also help you build your stabilization during compound exercises such and squats or deadlifts.

1. Sit on the edge of a bench and set the barbell on top of your legs. Measure your feet with your body so they're the same length apart as your shoulders.

2. With the palm of your hands facing down, grab the bar while keeping your hands at a wider distance than your shoulders.

3. Lift the bar up and over your head until your arms are extended fully.

4. Lower the bar behind you, letting it rest on the base of your neck. You're now at the starting position.

5. Move your torso from side to side but don't let other parts of your body, including your feet, move. You want to let your oblique muscles feel the contractions. Don't push your body to go further than what you're comfortable with because you can cause injury. Keep your movements controlled and slow. Every time you move to the side, exhale and then inhale when you bring your body back to the starting point.

6. Repeat this process for as many repetitions necessary in your set.

THE PERFECT PARTNERSHIP: BUNS AND THIGHS

After trying various upper body exercises, you can already start to feel the changes. You might even notice that your self-confidence is improving already and you're set to get started on your lower body.

GLUTES (THE PEACH)

There are three main muscles in your glute: gluteus minimus, gluteus maximus, and gluteus medius. The largest muscle is the gluteus maximus and its main function is moving the upper leg backwards, such as when you're rising from a squat. This muscle has a tendon at the end that connects to the hip muscles. The middle or medius muscle connects to the hip joint and works with the smallest glute muscle, the minimus, to help move your knee and hip joints. These are the muscles you'll work when you're extending your knee, flexing your hips, or running.

Back Extension (With Weight)

The main muscle that gets a workout with this exercise is the lower back. It also targets the glutes and hamstrings. You'll usually perform it on a 45 degree bench and have your feet anchored. You don't need to add a lot of weight to start working those muscles.

1. Lie face down on a hyperextension bench. Tuck your angles securely underneath the footpads to help you hold your proper form. If you need to adjust the pad, do so as you want your upper thighs to lie flat across the wide pad. You only need enough room to bend at the waist.
2. Keep your body straight and either place your arms behind your head or cross them in front of your chest. This is your starting position.
3. Keep your head neutral, inhale, and hinge your hips and lower your upper body toward the ground. Bend as far as you can go but keep your back straight.
4. Bring yourself back up to the starting point without moving your neck and keeping your back straight. It can help if you also inhale again as you bring yourself back up.
5. Repeat for the number of recommended repetitions.

Single-Leg Cable Hip Extension

This exercise focuses on the gluteus maximus but also targets the other two smaller muscles. It adds size and strength to your peach area and is great for lighter weights. The cable will help keep the muscles in a constant state of tension. You should perform between 8 to 12 repetitions in one set.

1. Begin by facing a low cable pulley and attach an ankle attachment around one ankle.
2. With a distance of about two feet between you and the weight stack, lean forward slightly and grab on to the machine to give you stability and help keep your proper form. This is your starting position.
3. Exhale and gradually kick your leg back while keeping your back and knee straight and your core tight. Hold this position for a couple of seconds so you can work the muscles well.
4. Inhale and bring your leg forward, back to the starting position. Repeat for the number of repetitions you set and then switch legs.

Barbell Hip Thrust

The hip thrust can be performed with or without barbells. If you've never tried this exercise before, it's best to do it without weights and then add them into your routine when you're ready. Because the weights sit across your midsection, it will build your glutes but also focus on your other leg muscles.

1. Sit down with a bench behind you.
2. Lean back a bit so your shoulder blades are near the top. Bend your knees and set the barbell across your lap. You're now at the starting position.
3. Press into your feet and balance your body at the edge of the bench to lift your hips off of the ground, keeping the weight balanced on your midsection. Exhale and ensure you squeeze your glutes so your knees and shoulders are aligned. Tuck in your chin so your neck is protected.
4. Exhale and slowly bring yourself back down close to the starting position. You don't want your hips to touch the floor until you're done with the repetitions.

Single-Leg Deadlifts

The main targets for this exercise are the gluteus muscles, but it also includes the calves and hamstrings. You can do this exercise at home if you have a kettlebell or any weight that you can grab by a handle so you don't need to worry about it sliding out of your hand or injuring yourself. You should do between 10 to 15 repetitions in each set.

1. Stand flat on the floor with a kettlebell in your left hand. This is your standing position.

2. Keeping your back straight and your neck neutral, inhale and gradually raise your left leg by hinging your hip and slightly bending your right knee. You want to get your leg up so your hips are squared forward and your shin is vertical. Try to keep your weight in your right foot, specifically between the heel and the midfoot.

3. Exhale and slowly bring your left leg back down to the standing position.

4. Repeat this process with as many repetitions as you set and then switch to the right leg.

QUADS

The quads or quadriceps are made up of four muscles: rectus femoris, vastus lateralis, vastus intermedius, and vastus medialis. Their main function is to help with knee movement, specifically with straightening. But they each have their own function as well.

The rectus femoris crosses at the knee and hip joint, which means it has two heads. It starts down at the front of your thigh and moves its way to your kneecap. The muscle helps with both knee extension and hip flexion.

The vastus lateralis is the largest of the four and it attaches from your patella to the top of your outer thigh. This is one of the muscles you want to focus on if you want to build and size up your thigh.

The muscle that sits deepest on your femur or thigh bone is the vastus intermedius. If you look at an anatomy image of these muscles, this one is partially covered by the rectus femoris. Its location is down the center of your thigh.

Running along the inside of your thigh is the vastus medialis. If you want to get that teardrop contour look above your knee, this is the muscle you want to focus on during your workout routine.

It's important to note that along with your back muscles, the quads are commonly injured in the gym due to tendonitis and muscle strains. This tends to happen when you move too fast during your workout or perform too many reps. Whenever you feel that you've strained a muscle, no matter where it is, you need to take time to let it heal or you can do more damage to it. Fortunately, most strains will heal on their own within a week.

Dumbbell Reverse Lunge

This is an exercise that some people like to perform instead of running or jogging for definition in the legs. It's friendly on your knees and helps you gain size and strengthen your quads along with the glutes, hamstrings, and hips. If you maintain the proper form, you can also build muscles in your lower back. It's almost like you're getting a full-body workout! It's best to focus on doing at least a dozen repetitions. It will also help you improve your core stability and flexibility.

If you find that your knees have trouble with this exercise, then you want to focus on squats because you'll get similar results.

1. While holding a dumbbell in each hand, rest them on your sides and stand up straight. This is your starting position.
2. Inhale and step back with one leg. Set your toes on the floor behind you and lower yourself down. Keep your back straight and your head neutral. Both of your knees should be at a 90 degree angle with your back knee under your hip and your front knee directly above your ankle.
3. Exhale and then bring yourself back to the starting position gradually by stepping on your back foot, bringing it forward. To give your quads the best workout, use the ball of your feet to push.
4. Repeat these steps with the opposite leg.
5. Complete your set with your number of repetitions.

Lying Leg Curls

You'll need to use a machine to perform this exercise, but it's a common one so you should find it easily in the gym. It's a great beginner's exercise because it helps build and size up your quads, glutes, and calves. You will usually do about a dozen repetitions in one set, if not more.

1. Make sure to adjust the machine lever so it fits your height before you lay face down on it. The key is to place the pad of the level just a few inches under your calves. If you want to build your hamstrings more within the workout, you'll want to angle the machine downward so your head is lower to the ground. Otherwise, you can leave the machine flat.
2. With your torso flat on the bench and your head in a neutral position, stretch out your legs fully and grab the handles of the machine. This will help you keep the proper form. Position your toes so they are straight. You are now at the starting position.
3. Exhale and curl your legs up, pushing the pad at your ankles. Without lifting your upper legs, push up as far as you can. When you've reached your upwards position, hold yourself there for a couple of seconds.
4. Inhale and bring your legs down to the starting position gradually.
5. Repeat for the number of repetitions for your set.

Machine (Hack) Squat

There are many ways you can perform a squat. One of the main ways to strengthen your quads is through the machine squat. You'll also build your hamstrings and glutes. When using the machine, you want to stick at least 12 to 15 repetitions in one set.

1. Lay face up on a hack squat machine and ensure your shoulders are securely placed underneath the shoulder pads.

2. Place your feet on the platform with your toes slightly pointed out and at shoulder-length distance.

3. Set your arms on the side handles and straighten out your body but don't lock your knees. You're now at the starting position.

4. Keeping your back straight and your neck neutral, inhale, and slowly bend your knees to lower the machine. Keep going down until you have about a 90 degree angle between your calves and upper leg or until the calves are parallel to the floor. The front of your knees should be straight with your toes. If you're beyond this point you went too far and you can create stress on your body, which can cause injury.

5. Exhale and gradually rise by pushing the platform with the heels of your foot until you're back in the starting position.

6. Repeat this exercise for your recommended number of repetitions.

Narrow Leg Press

This exercise is similar to a machine squat but it's reversed and often with more weight. It focuses on your quads, but will also strengthen your calves and hamstrings. You should complete between 8 to 12 repetitions in one set.

1. Lay your torso on the pad so your back is straight and your neck is neutral. Position your hands on the grips to help you keep the proper form.
2. Set your feet on the platform with your heels at the bottom and keep them about shoulder width apart. This is your starting position.
3. Keeping your back straight and without lifting yourself off the set, exhale and press the platform up until your legs are almost straight but don't lock your knees.
4. Inhale and gradually bring the platform back down.
5. Repeat for as many repetitions needed in your set.

HAMSTRINGS

The main muscles in the hamstrings include the semimembranosus, semitendinosus, and biceps femoris. They are located on the back of the thigh and they link the knee joint to the pelvis. If you want to feel them, stand up straight and then push your leg behind you; this is your hamstring and glutes at work. The procedure is called a hip extension. If you lift one heel toward your glutes while standing, you're performing a knee flexion.

The hamstrings help you bend your knee and extend your leg straight back. When you focus on building them up, you will spend your time with knee and hip exercises.

You've already learned about many exercises that improve the strength of your hamstrings, but there are a few more to add to your routine.

Reverse Hyperextension

You will use a machine to help build your hamstrings with the reverse hyperextension. You can use different weight amounts but also gain good strength with light weight.

1. Set your feet between the pads and lay your hips on the torso pad so they are hanging off of it. Grab the handles and lift yourself up a bit so you can hold the position. Your feet will hang down while securely sitting between the pads. This is your starting position.
2. Flex your hips so you're pulling your legs forward.
3. Reverse the motion so you're extending your hips and legs, like you're kicking your legs back. Perform this movement gradually so you don't overextend your hips as this can cause injury. You want to stop right before you reach your full range motion.
4. Move your legs forward again, going as far as you can underneath the equipment.
5. Repeat for the necessary amount of repetitions you set.

Smith Machine Squat

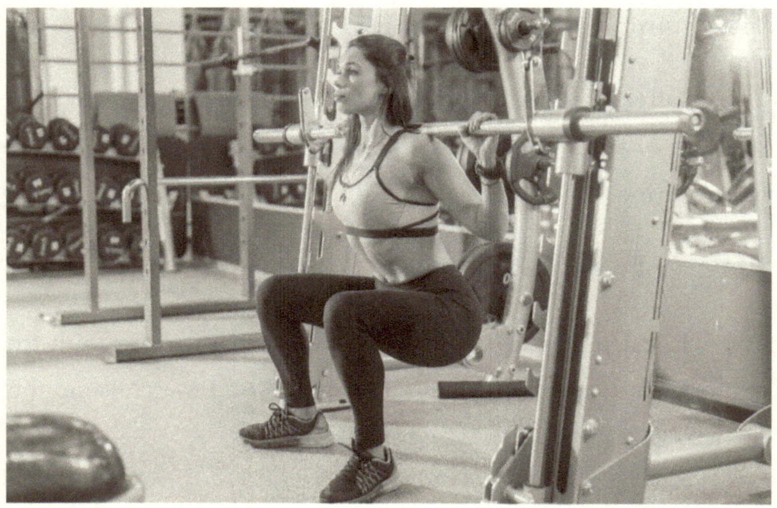

The Smith machine mimics the barbells but gives you more stability which can help beginners hold their proper form easier. This exercise is often part of a lower-body and full-body workout because it adds strength and size to your glutes, hamstrings, and quads. You should perform between 8 to 12 repetitions in each set.

1. Begin by placing the bar at the machine height that matches your size. Once you're ready, step underneath the bar and place it slightly below your neck and on the back of your shoulders.

2. With your palms facing forward, hold the bar securely on both sides at a wider width than your shoulders.

3. Unlock the bar from the machine and push it out with your legs while straightening your torso.

4. Slightly point your toes out and move your legs so there is about the same width between them as your shoulders. You're now in the starting position.

5. Inhale and push your hips back while bending your knees. Lower your body until your thighs are at or a bit below parallel, about 90 degrees.

6. Let your knees track over your toes while keeping your head neutral and your back straight.

7. Exhale as you push yourself back up by putting much of the weight in your heels. Extend to back to the starting position.

8. Repeat for the number of repetitions you set for yourself.

Seated Leg Curl

This is similar to the lying leg curl but it can feel a bit more challenging. It will not only build your hamstrings but also strengthen your glutes, though to a lesser degree. If you're having trouble with squats or deadlift exercises, this is a great way to help strengthen your legs so you can perform these workouts correctly. You should include between 8 to 12 repetitions per set.

1. Sit on a leg curl machine with your back straight on the back rest. Rest your ankles on top of the pad. Grab

the handles to help stability and keep your focus on your hamstrings. This is your starting position.

2. Exhale and curl your knees back toward your hips by pushing down on the pad. Keep your back against the seat and your core tight.

3. Inhale and gradually extend your legs back to the starting position.

4. Repeat for as many repetitions that are in your set.

Barbell Good Morning

Along with targeting the hamstrings, this exercise also aims for the glutes and lower back. Because of the weight you put on your lower back and how damaging this can be over time, especially if you fall away from proper form, keep the repetitions to under eight in one set.

1. Place a barbell over the back of your shoulder with your palms facing forward. Stand tall so your back is straight, your shoulder blades pinched together, and your neck is neutral. This is your starting position.

2. Breathe in and hinge your hips to bend forward while keeping your back straight. Bend your knees slightly to help keep your balance.

3. Breathe out and push your weight into your heel to help your glutes engage so you can start slowly bringing yourself back to starting position.

4. Repeat for the recommended number of repetitions.

CALVES

If you're sitting down and you've been sitting for a while, get up —not only because it's not good to sit for over 45 minutes, but because it's time to get up on your toes. Stretch to help yourself feel your muscles. Do you notice that you feel your calves more than other muscles? This is because what you just did is called a calf raise. Yes, it's a minor stretch and exercise that you can perform to help build your calves.

There are two main muscles in your calves, the soleus and the gastrocnemius. The soleus is located underneath and is in action the most when you're walking and standing. The gastrocnemius is the one you use when you're jumping and running. It will bunch up when flexed because it has two heads.

Seated Calf Raise

You already did a brief standing calf raise so now it's time to look at the seated position. This is used with a machine and focuses mainly on the soleus muscle. You should perform between 8 to 12 repetitions at minimum.

1. Sit down on the machine with your toes on the steps and your thighs under the pads. This is your starting position.
2. Exhale and press down with your toes to make your calf muscles work and raise your heels. Keep your back straight, chest up, and neck neutral.

3. Inhale and slowly bring yourself back to the starting position.

4. Repeat these steps for the number of repetitions you decide.

Barbell Seated Calf Raise

Now that you have an idea (or tried) the seated calf raise without weight, it's time to include weights.

1. Sit down at the edge of a bench with a box that's about a foot tall in front of you.

2. Set the ball of your feet on the box with your heels hanging off. Make sure your feet are flat.

3. Place a barbell about three inches above your knees and hold it there with the palms of your hands pointing down. This is your starting position.

4. While squeezing your calves, raise your toes up as much as you can. Exhale when you perform this step.

5. Hold the contraction for a second or two then inhale and bring yourself back to the starting position.

6. Repeat for about 8 to 12 repetitions.

Weighted Donkey Calf Raise

This exercise is used with a weighted donkey calf machine. It mainly focuses on the gastrocnemius muscle. If you're beginning to learn this routine, you want to focus on five to eight repetitions. Once you've gained muscle and experience, you will go up to a dozen in one set.

1. Wearing a weight belt, stand behind a low stool or box with a smaller step behind you.
2. Bend forward and place your hands on the box. Then, place your toes on the step and straighten your back. Keep your legs straight and let the weight hang down. This is your starting position.
3. Breath out and press yourself up with your toes while raising your heels so your calves are engaged.
4. Breathe in a lower yourself back to the starting position slowly as you continue to keep your neck neutral and your back straight.
5. Repeat this process for the number of recommended repetitions.

Smith Machine Reverse Calf Raise

To build and size up your calves, you want to focus on this exercise. It's performed with a machine and is great for a beginner because you feel the benefits with little weight. You should include about 8 to 12 repetitions in your set.

1. Fit the barbell on the machine to your height.
2. Set a raised platform directly underneath the bar and stand on it with your heels on and the balls of your feet off the edge.

3. Face your toes forward and keep them at a shoulder-length distance.

4. Grab the barbell with your palms facing forward and lean it against the back of your shoulders.

5. Extend your hips and knees to push up on the barbell so your torso is standing straight up but your knees are slightly bent. You want to keep them from locking. You're now at the starting position.

6. Exhale and raise the balls of your feet. Flex your calf by extending your toes as high as you can. You should not bend your knees or any other part of your body at any time. Keep your back straight and your neck neutral. Hold this position for a couple of seconds.

7. Inhale and gradually bring yourself back to the starting point.

8. Repeat for the number of recommendations in your set.

THE PERFECT PANDEMIC PROOF PLAN: BUILD TONED MUSCLE AT HOME

You're confident about heading to the gym after learning a few great workouts to perform with proper form. You know that you can walk in there with your head held high. You don't see the looks from other people as a negative because it doesn't matter to you. While you still need to learn and grow (you should never stop), this doesn't mean you don't belong at the gym—it means that you're perfect for it. But this still doesn't stop you from wondering, "How can I build my muscles at home?" It happens in the busy world you live in. You can't get to the gym because of the weather, long days at work, and those unexpected moments where your children are sick or surprise you with a school performance. Maybe you want to get your children or partner to work out with you at home so they'll think about joining the gym with you. There might also be a lockdown when gyms are closed and you're told to stay at home.

You already know that there are a variety of exercises you can do at home, such as running, push-ups, crunches, and squats. Well, you must think this is a short list, but it's not all the work-outs you can complete. In fact, let's look at a variety of exercises you can perform within a few minutes to a couple of full body workouts!

BUILD MUSCLES WITHOUT WEIGHTS AT HOME

Balance Board

If you feel that you have trouble with your balance during your exercises, this is a great step to take to build a weakness. It doesn't include weights, but does use a specific board that you stand on and move around as there is a round piece underneath. You can move yourself in a circle motion, side to side, or front to back. Use your hands and arms to help you learn how to balance but keep your body straight the whole time as this will also allow you to focus on your form. There are a number of balancing boards, so if you have trouble with one, you can try a different type.

1. Place the board in front of you and stand on it.
2. Have your feet a few inches apart to give you the best form while keeping your back straight and neck neutral.
3. Hold your balance for as long as you feel necessary.

Because you're standing and keeping your balance, you are strengthening your calves.

Back Extension (Without Weight)

The back extension exercise will help you build your glutes and hamstrings. It also increases your muscular endurance and lower back strength. You can perform it on a stability ball, also known as an exercise or Yoga ball. You've probably seen one dozens of times as they're used in several exercises. Other ways are on a 45-degree bench with your feet anchored or a mat so you can complete it at home or at the gym. Usually, you will complete at least 8 to 12 reps during each set if using weight. If you're not using weight, such as with the ball, you'll perform at least 15 to 20 reps.

1. Start by lying face down on a hyperextension bench or a stability ball. If you're using a bench, which beginners find easier, you'll tuck your ankles under the foot pads. If you're using a ball, place your hands behind your head and feet under a stable piece of furniture that you won't lift up or tip over.
2. Adjust yourself if necessary, such as ensuring that your upper thighs lie across the wide bar in a comfortable position so you're not squirming or losing your form while exercising. On the machine, you can place your hands behind your head or cross them above over your chest.

3. Keep your body straight with your arms and feet in place. This is your starting position.

4. Bend forward slowly at your waist, bringing yourself as far as you can and until you feel your hamstring stretch. Keep your back straight the whole time and inhale as you perform this portion of the exercise.

5. Once you feel the stretch, exhale as you raise your body up with your back straight and arms in place. Gradually bring yourself back to your starting position. Don't swing your torso as you can injure your back.

6. Continue this process for the number of repetitions you're set on.

Scissor Kick

The scissor kick will help you work on your lower abs. Like crunches, you'll lie straight on your back but have your legs up a little and rotate your legs up and down. You should do at least 10 to 15 reps in each set.

1. Extend your arms fully out on each side while you're lying down. Keep your palms facing down.

2. Lift your legs up so your heels are about five to six inches from the floor and bend your knees slightly. You're now in the starting position.

3. Lower your right leg until it's about two to three inches from the ground as you lift your left leg up to a 45 degree angle.

4. Reverse the position of your legs without them touching the ground or the rest of your body, including your arms, moving.

5. Repeat until you're done with the set.

Exercise Ball Leg Curl

You will usually use your bodyweight for this exercise. It will build and strengthen your hamstring muscles and your glutes. If you can't get to a lying leg curl machine, this is a great substitute. You will need an exercise ball.

1. Lie on your back with your arms on the side and your lower legs resting on an exercise ball. You want to ensure that the ball is in a position so when you lift up, your ankles will move to the top of the ball. You can practice a bit before you start the exercise to get the right feel. Once you have the sweet spot, this is your starting position.

2. Lift your hips off the ground by using your glutes.

3. Keeping your core engaged, bend your knees to roll the ball in while keeping your back as straight as possible while it rises and your feet firmly on the ball.

4. Your neck and head should stay on the floor along with your arms.

5. Gradually extend your legs by rolling the ball away from under you and close to the starting position but don't let your hips touch the floor.

6. Repeat for the rest of your repetitions.

Crunches

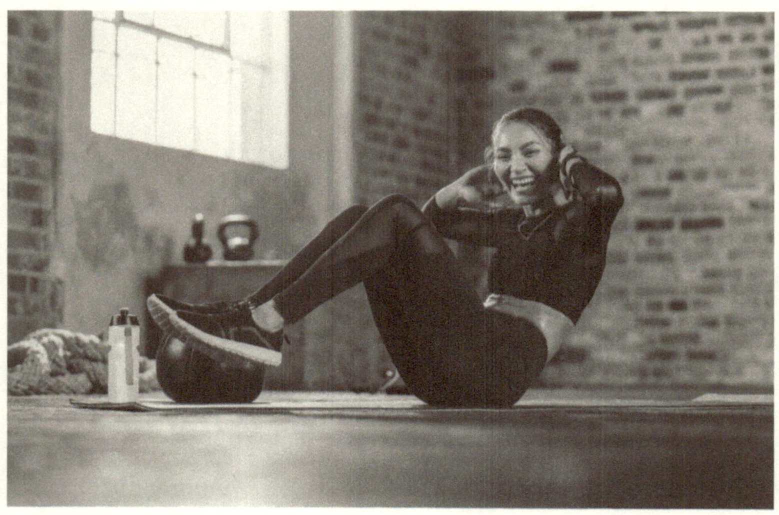

One of the most popular exercises to help build your upper abs are crunches, which are often confused with sit ups. Crunches don't go all the way up to your knees whereas sit ups will. Plus, you tend to go faster and you generally have your hands behind your head for the best form. Your feet can be unanchored or anchored to the floor, sometimes you'll have someone or furniture help keep your feet firmly down.

1. Lie your back flat on the floor and your knees bent. Keep your feet flat on the floor and put your fingers behind your ears. This is your starting position.

2. Exhale and lift your shoulder blades to contract your abs while pressing your lower back into the floor. Don't use momentum and raise your upper body slowly while keeping the rest of your body as still as possible.

3. Gradually lower your shoulder blacks back down to the starting position while you inhale.

4. Repeat this process for as many repetitions in your set.

Rear Leg Raises

These are exercises that you can use with just your bodyweight or a stretch band to give your muscles more of a workout. There are many muscles in your leg that will feel this workout, but the main one is the quadriceps.

1. Start by placing a mat on the floor (optional) and then get yourself on your hands and knees. So you don't damage your body, it's best to have something softer underneath you if you're on a hard floor.

2. Your head is down, looking at the back of your hands, while your shoulders are facing forward. Your knees should be bent at a 90 degree angle. You're now at your starting position.

3. Lift your left leg up behind you, extending both your knee and hip. Get your leg as straight as possible with your foot high above your head. Hold this position for

a second before lowering it back down to the starting
position.

4. Repeat for five to ten repetitions with the left leg
   before switching to the right.

FULL BODY WORKOUT 1

This routine is completed in about 15 minutes and all you need
is one light dumbbell, between 3 to 8 pounds, and one heavier
dumbbell, between 10 to 15 pounds. Each exercise should be
performed at least 10 to 12 times. You can add a few more reps
but don't push yourself too much so you don't strain your
muscles. You also want to repeat the set a couple of times (so
think of this when setting your number of reps). It's best to
complete it three to five times a week.

Squat to Shoulder Press

1. Stand on your mat with your feet wider than shoulder
   width apart.
2. Put a heavier weight in each hand and hold them near
   your shoulders. You should have the palms of your
   hands pointing toward you. This is your starting
   position.
3. Squat down while keeping your back straight and your
   head neutral.
4. Bring yourself back up by pushing the weight into your
   heels to get back to your standing position.

5. Raise your arms straight up while keeping the rest of your body in position.

6. Bring your arms back down to the starting point.

7. Repeat this exercise for as many repetitions that you set before taking a short break and going to the next workout.

Lunge to Single-Arm Row

1. Put a heavier barbell in your right hand. On your mat, move your left leg forward with the knee bent slightly. Push your right leg back until it is extended but don't lock your knee. Keep your back and neck straight so it makes a diagonal line with your right leg. Set your left hand against your left thigh. This is your starting position.

2. Lunge down by bending both knees and keeping your right arm down so the barbell is close to the height of your left ankle.

3. Slowly bring your legs back into starting position but raise your elbow so it draws closer to the ceiling. Keep the elbow close to your body.

4. When you bring yourself back down, lower the weight back down toward the floor.

5. Repeat this repetition between 10 to 12 times and then switch sides.

Deadlift to Bicep Curl

1. Step on your mat with a dumbbell in each hand. Stand with your feet shoulder width apart. This is your starting position.
2. Squat down but keep the weights close to your shins. Most the palms of your hands so they're facing your shins. You will do a little movement in your wrists as you bend down, slowly twist them from the side of your legs to the front.
3. Gradually bring yourself back up to starting position then hinge your elbows to raise the weights to your shoulders. The palm of your hand should point toward your body. Bring the weights down to the starting point.
4. Repeat for 8 to 10 repetitions.

Curtsy Lunge to Upright Row

1. With a light dumbbell in each hand, step on the mat, keeping your feet about shoulder width apart. This is your starting position.
2. Moving your right foot, step back to the left. Bend your right knee to curtsy while letting the barbells lower close to your knee. Keep your back straight and your head neutral.
3. Step back into the starting point and then bend your

elbows into an upright row so the weights are hanging near your chest. The palms of your hands should be pointing behind you.

4. Then move your left foot back to the right. Bend your left knee to curtsy, keeping the barbells closer to your knee like before.

5. Repeat this process for 10 to 12 repetitions.

Bridge to Headbanger

1. With a dumbbell in each hand, lie down on your back with your legs bent. Extend your arms toward the ceiling with your palms facing each other. This is your starting position.

2. Squeeze your glutes to lift up your hips while pressing the weight into your feet to form a bridge.

3. Bend your elbows and slowly bring the weights down by your ears while holding the bridge by squeezing your glutes. Keep your upper back, neck, and head on the floor.

4. Gradually bring yourself back to the starting point.

5. Repeat this exercise between 10 to 12 times.

Russian Twist into a Pike

1. Sit down on your mat and bend your knees.
2. Lean back and lift your feet off the floor so your legs are extended and you're balancing on your glutes.
3. Lower your legs and place your hands in a position so it looks like they're holding a ball in front of you. Extend your arms.
4. Twist your torso to the left and then the right while keeping your knees bent and your back straight. Twist your torso in the same manner again. Bring your arms back to the center and extend as you extend your legs.
5. Repeat this exercise between 10 to 12 times.

Push-up to Plank Jack

1. Get on your hands and knees and then lift yourself up so you're supported by the palm of your hands and the ball of your feet. Your hands are directly under your shoulders. This is your starting position, also known as the plank.
2. Lower yourself into a push-up while bending your elbows.
3. Bring yourself back up to the plank.
4. Jump your feet so you spread them apart to the side like you would a jumping jack. Bring yourself back into the starting position.

5. Repeat this exercise for 10 to 12 times.

FULL BODY WORKOUT 2

This full body workout can be completed in about 20 to 25 minutes. You should always take a little break between each exercise and make sure to drink enough water so you don't get dehydrated. All you will need are a pair of dumbbells, a mat, and some music if it helps you kick your motivation into high gear.

Glute Bridge

1. Lay down on your back and bend your knees. Let your arms rest by your sides with the palms toward the floor. Have your feet flat on the floor and keep them the same width as your hips. This is your starting position.
2. Squeeze your abs and glutes so you can lift your hips and lower back up while pushing through your heels. Keep your feet flat and don't move your upper back, neck, head, or arms. Raise yourself up until your body forms a straight line from your shoulders to your knees. Hold this position for a couple of seconds.
3. Gradually bring your body back down to the starting position.
4. Repeat this exercise for 30 seconds before taking a five second break and moving on.

Dead Bug

1. Lay down on your back (like the name suggests) and extend your arms up toward the ceiling.
2. Bring your legs up but bend at your knees so they're in a tabletop position. Your knees should be above your hips and your legs in a 90 degree position. This is your starting point.
3. Slowly bring your left arm overhead, keeping it straight, so it's like you're stretching above your head. At the same time, you want to extend your right leg so it's straight out, just a few inches from the floor, but don't lock your knee.
4. Bring your arm and leg back into starting position and repeat the procedure with your opposite leg and arm.
5. Continue for 30 seconds before taking a five second break.

Bird Dog

1. Get down on your hands and knees. Keep your palms to the floor and your back straight. You want your neck to be in a neutral position. This is your starting point.
2. Straighten out your left leg and extend your right arm at the same time. Keep them in a straight line with your body for a couple of seconds.

3. Gradually bring them back to the starting position and then repeat the process with your other leg and arm.

4. Repeat this exercise for 30 seconds and then take a five second break.

Bodyweight Squat

1. Begin by standing with your feet shoulder width apart.

2. You can place your hands behind your back or head. This is your starting position. If you're holding a bar you want to put it behind your head, resting on the back of your neck. You will have your palms facing the ceiling.

3. Inhale and bend your knees as you start pushing your hips back. Lower yourself like you're about to sit on a chair until your thighs are below or parallel with your knees. Keep your weight in your heels and your torso upright. You can bring your hands folded out in front of you as you move down to help you balance.

4. Exhale and reverse back to starting position by keeping your torso straight and your head up. Push your knees out and use your heels to help bring yourself back up.

5. Repeat this exercise for 30 seconds and then take a minute break.

Squat to Overhead Press

1. With a dumbbell in each hand, stand with your feet slightly wider than your shoulders and hips.
2. Hinge your elbows so the weights are parallel to your shoulders. Keep your palms facing in and your back straight. Your head should be neutral. This is your starting position.
3. Get into a squat position by bending your knees and pushing your hips back. Ensure you don't move the position of your back or neck.
4. Raise yourself back up to starting position but once you get there, lift your arms over your head until they're fully extended.
5. Gradually lower your arms back to the starting point.
6. Repeat this exercise for 30 seconds before taking a 15 second break.

Bent Over Row

1. Holding a weight in each hand, keep your arms on your sides with your palms toward your body.
2. Move your feet so they're about the same lengths as between your hips.
3. Engage your core and hinge your hips forward so your glutes are pushed back. Slightly bend your knees but keep your back straight and your chest out.

4. Keeping your elbows close to your body, bring the weights up by bending your elbows toward the ceiling, similar to rowing a boat. Once the weights are near your chest, squeeze your shoulder muscles for a couple of seconds.

5. Slowly lower the weights by extending your arms back to their starting position.

6. Repeat this process for 30 seconds before a 15 second break.

Wood Chop

1. Stand up straight and move your feet so they're wider than hip length apart.

2. Hold a dumbbell with both hands near your left leg and engage your core.

3. Diagonally raise your arms in front of your body, bringing the weight from your left leg up above your right shoulder. Do not twist your wrists or move your hands. You want to twist your body with the dumbbell but keep your back straight and your neck neutral. Allow your toes to naturally rotate.

4. Now bring the weight down or "chop" it by reversing your movement and bringing the barbell back toward the left side of your body. Do not bend your arms, always keep them extended.

5. Continue for 15 seconds and then switch sides and

perform for another 15 seconds. Then, take a break for one minute.

V-Ups

1. Lie down on your back. Extend your arms so they're over your head, a bit above the floor. You can hold your hands out so your thumbs are touching the floor but keep your arms close to your ears. Extend your legs as well. You're now at the starting position.
2. Point your toes, squeeze your glutes and thighs together.
3. Lift your upper back off the ground while keeping it straight. Don't break the extension of your arms. Allow them to help lift you up. Simultaneously, lift your legs but keep them straight.
4. Bring your arms and legs together until they are parallel with each other while keeping your core engaged. Your body will form a "v" shape.
5. Slowly bring yourself back to the starting position.
6. Continue this exercise for 30 seconds and take a 15 second break.

Up and Down Plank

1. Get down on your hands and knees. Place the palms of your hands on the floor and keep your back straight. Your hands should be at shoulder width apart. Your shoulders and wrists should be stacked against your day.

2. Extend your legs behind you. Keep your glutes and core engaged to keep a flat back and avoid a rounding back or sinking stomach. Set your feet so they are hip width apart. You're now in the starting position.

3. Lower your right arm so that your forearm is lying on the floor. Repeat the same motion with your left arm while keeping your back straight and your neck in a neutral position. You're now in the plank setting.

4. Slowly lift yourself up, right arm and then left, back to the starting point. Keep your hips as still as you can so you don't start swaying them.

5. Continue this process for 30 seconds.

8

CONSISTENCY, CONSISTENCY, CONSISTENCY!

You've been there before—you wake up to your alarm and think, "I don't need exercise today because I did it yesterday. Sleep is more important." While sleep is important, so is staying consistent with your daily schedule and workout routine. If you set a goal to head to the gym before work five days a week, then you need to get up and go to the gym. Yes, there will be days where you don't feel like getting up. There are also days where you don't feel well. But, you need to stop your sudden thoughts of "I don't need to exercise today" and head to the gym.

Obviously you do not need to get up and move when you're sick or an emergency pops up. Life happens and sometimes you can't stick to your schedule. However, you can't let excuses get in your way because this leads you to an inconsistent workout routine and mindset, which brings you down the road to sitting in your car at the McDonald's drive-thru and realizing you haven't been to the gym in close to a week. Okay, maybe this is a bit far-fetched but you understand the point.

THREE KEYS TO CONSISTENCY

The point is you need to remain consistent as much as possible. It's understandable that you may feel a bit impatient when it comes to working out. Unfortunately, your body won't change overnight. You might start feeling the workout, but you won't see results right away. To reap the benefits that you're looking for, you need to work at it regularly for months. You need to follow the diet and the exercise routine that you set up for yourself. If you don't stick to it consistently, you will feel like you're spinning your wheels but not getting anywhere, and this is frustrating. You can't get your curves while sitting in a parked car.

1. Resistance Training improves your muscular strength and is sometimes referred to as strength training or weight training. When you exercise, you focus on moving your body against resistance, making it harder to perform. For example, using dumbbells with added weight or moving your body against gravity. The main benefits are that you'll not only start to lose weight, but also get tighter, leaner, and stronger.

Remember, it's best to start with weight that you're comfortable with or that you can handle well and get used to good form and then add a few pounds every time you want to increase your weight.

2. *Cardiovascular Training* is perfect for the days where you can't just bring yourself to lifting weights. Hey, it will happen, even when you feel the benefits and you're proud of the curves you've received. When you feel that weight lifting is a lifestyle and you'll never go back, you will have days where you look at the weights and equipment and go, "I'm just not feeling it today." You can even try to boost your motivation through techniques and still find yourself struggling. Instead of trying to force yourself to lift, look at taking a quick, little break and turning to cardio. One of two steps can happen. First, you'll find the motivation for strength training at the end of your workout. Two, you'll be proud of yourself for working out and find that you're ready to go back to lifting the next day.

You never want to ignore cardiovascular training. It will help boost your metabolism and burn a few extra calories. It will help you lose weight and stay in shape, especially when connected to weight lifting. You can start your workout routine by doing cardio exercises right away in the morning and then move into lifting, or you can do it immediately after weight training to help yourself find a more relaxed state. This is usually a better system to use if you find yourself working out before you head to bed.

3. Nutrition is probably where the biggest inconsistency is, at least for most people. You start to miss certain foods that you need to limit or you tell yourself that you can't consume. There is the belief that a "cheat day" helps you stick to a diet when it takes you away from the consistency. You also find yourself struggling to know what to eat when you go out to a restaurant with your family or friends, or to the movies. I know how it goes. Those two bags of candy are calling your name, telling you they were made specifically for you. Don't worry, I've been there too. The reality is, once you set your diet you need to maintain consistency so you don't start losing your mindset. You want to moderate yourself because this is a true key. It's okay to have a little butter on your popcorn, as long as you don't indulge yourself for two hours. Keep in mind the diet you set up earlier, using a variety of healthy foods, and stick to it consistently.

TIPS TO STAY MOTIVATED

Connect with friends or a personal trainer. To gain more dedication, you look for a personal training or a workout partner. You might find someone in the gym that can help keep you accountable with your exercise routine or talk one of your friends into a gym membership. They can also give you motivation by being your cheerleader, make you follow your workout plan, and brainstorm with you when you find yourself getting bored with the same exercises. Plus, working out with someone just makes the process more fun, even when you're sweating.

Set goals you can attain. You have an ideal body that you want but this doesn't mean you can reach it quickly or easily. It's easy to put your perfect body image in your mind and forget about certain basics, such as your bone structure. You want to get an idea of the curves you want for your body and not what you see walking down the red carpet during the Golden Globes or in a magazine. You need to be realistic and set goals that you can achieve. For instance, if you want to lose 50 pounds within the year, start by stating your goal in a way that gives you motivation. You might say, "By this time next year I will have lost 50 pounds." Then, you want to establish steps to help you lose the weight. How many pounds will you lose every month? Can you look at losing four to five pounds every month? If you believe this is attainable through your workout routine and diet, set your mind to it.

Practice mindfulness. Your mind is meant to focus on two levels of awareness: mindfulness and mindlessness. You're usually stuck in a mindless trance where you're going through your daily motions. You know your drive to work so you get lost in your thoughts and don't pay close attention to the road until you get to your destination and think, "I don't remember going through this neighborhood or passing that building." You pick up your kids from school or daycare, make dinner, and complete chores without much thought. When it comes to staying motivated, mindlessness is a problem because it can lead to boredom. You can also forget about your form and seriously hurt yourself during your routine.

Mindfulness is the opposite. It's knowing what you're thinking, doing, and how you're feeling. You're aware of your body's sensations and mind to muscle connection so you know when it's enough weight, when to bend, lift, where your arms, and legs should be. There is also an art to being mindful and that's living in the moment. You're not worried about paying bills, what you need to do when you get home, or how stressed you feel. Instead, you're focusing on you. You're giving yourself time to do what you want to do so you can better yourself and this is an important part of your day. In fact, you'll start to look forward to it because you can release your stress and escape from the busyness of life.

Make working out a part of your day. You have a daily routine from the time you get up to when you go to bed. Sometimes you're thrown a curve ball and need to go with the flow, but most days you know what you're supposed to do. For example, you need to get your kids ready, make sure lunches are made, get yourself ready for work, run errands, cook, clean, and so much more. Most of these steps you do because you're motivated, whether you feel like it or not. You want to give your children the best education so you ensure they get to school. You're determined to get your family to eat right so you cook healthy meals. You can consistently work out every day by adding it into your routine. Pick a certain time, such as before or after work, to stop at the gym or head down to your basement to lift weight and get some cardio done. You'll find that this helps you maintain a better mindset when it comes to exercises and soon you might find it a regular part of your routine, just like cooking healthy meals.

Don't forget the pep talk. Sometimes you need to be your own cheerleader. You need to get in front of the mirror and tell yourself, "You are doing great. You are looking good. You're losing weight and you're getting your curves. You got this. Keep it up. Do it." Whether the positivity comes from your workout buddy or yourself, it'll help keep you motivated. Even if you tell yourself, "I got this" before you walk to your equipment, you're giving yourself an emotional pep talk that can lead you to a great workout.

Eat often. You know that it's better to eat smaller meals more often throughout the day, so eat around the time you exercise. It doesn't matter if you have a small breakfast before or after, the key is to ensure that you have energy for your workout. For example, you might decide to eat every three hours so you prepare your meals ahead of time. The night before you sort out your snacks and side dishes, such as a salad, fruits, vegetables, and nuts. You put together your meals to the best of your abilities by making the wrap or cutting up the chicken to brown before your lunch. You might also add a few little extra snacks just in case something throws you off course by including to-go almond butter and Greek yogurt. It's also a good idea to plan your family's meals. This gives you the motivation to go home and warm up or cook the evening meal instead of stopping at a restaurant for a quick bite.

Remember how you feel after the workout. Most people say one of their biggest motivators to exercise is the way they feel afterwards. Some state that it's the way their muscles feel, even if they're a bit sore because they challenged themselves. It shows them that they worked hard and they're improving their body. Other people say that they like the way it mentally and emotionally makes them feel, gives them motivation for the rest of the day and makes them feel like they can take on the world. Taking a minute or two to think about how good you feel after your workout routine can give you the drive to hit the gym.

Surround yourself with the right people. The people you know are a great source of motivation, especially if they want you to succeed. Even though they might not have a plan to start exercising, they tell you how good you look, talk about how much you've changed, and how proud they are of you. All of the positive reinforcements they provide give you strength to continue working out. You can think about the positive statements they've made or give them a call when you're struggling to start training. They want you to reach your goals so they will support you and do what they can to help you through the tough moments.

CONCLUSION

Take a moment to feel your muscles. They're now building and strengthening. The more you stay consistent with your plan, the sooner you'll start to see the curves that you want. You started this journey by learning the five biggest benefits for weight training, such as boosting self-confidence, building curves in the right area, reducing stress and anxiety, burning more calories than fat, and finding your fountain of youth.

You then went on to learn about the difference between weight training and cardio. You discovered how many benefits are the same, but some are different. You also learned how you can include cardio into your workout routine to get the best results. From there, you found out that you can still eat some of your favorite foods, as long as you follow your healthy diet with basic nutrition and when you should eat.

You discovered how to walk into the gym like you own it. There is no need to worry about the stares you perceive you are receiving from people because you know what you're doing and you're doing a great job. You know all about proper form and how to pick exercises that are good for you. Plus, you received a variety of exercises in a step by step format from your upper body to lower. Of course, you also have two full body workouts that you can do at home.

One of the key takeaways is that you will now start to feel confident about your workout routine, whether at the gym or home. You will use proper form to keep yourself from injury and make you feel more comfortable with your exercises. You will start to feel that people who are looking in your direction are asking, "How does she do it? She looks so good" instead of thinking they are questioning you.

Another takeaway is that you learned how many repetitions so you do in each set. For example, you will usually keep them between 8 to 12 and do about 2 to 3 sets. Remember to take a short break between each set, which is a perfect time to take a drink of water.

You should also take away what exercises are best for you, whether at home or the gym. You know to focus on the muscles you want to tone and shape for your best curves. But, it's also important to focus on other parts of your body so you'll develop a routine that works best for you and then re-evaluate after a couple of months.

Another key takeaway is you know how to help yourself stay motivated. There will always be days you wonder if you need to go to the gym and the answer is that you don't because you have a full body workout you can perform at home! Along with this, you know how to apply the exercise into your schedule so you can make time to workout without letting several days go by and not exercise.

Now that you have everything you need to get the body you want, it's time to take action and develop your workout routine. Go out there and show everyone at the gym that you got this! Maybe you'll also help other women learn how they can own the gym through these simple and direct exercises.

I hope you enjoyed this book as much as I enjoyed writing it for you. Please leave a review on Amazon so you can help other women develop their curves and find confidence to enter the gym and eat right.

REFERENCES

Bodybuilding.com. (2015). Jessie hilgenberg's 6 reasons women should lift - bodybuilding.com [YouTube Video]. In YouTube. https://www.youtube.com/watch?v=e_zKn7H3v4w

Clark, S. (2016, July 20). Glute workout: 6 ways to build your perfect booty. Bodybuilding.Com. https://www.bodybuilding.com/content/glute-workout-6-ways-to-build-your-perfect-booty.html

Corleone, J. (2020, March 11). Weight-Training diet plan for women. LIVESTRONG.COM. https://www.livestrong.com/article/185048-weight-training-diet-plan-for-women/

Cornish, J. L. (2018, August 24). Shoulder workouts for women: 4 workouts to build size and shape. Bodybuilding.Com. https://www.bodybuilding.com/content/shoulder-workouts-for-women-4-workouts-to-build-size-and-shape.html

Cornish, J. L. (2019, August 12). Back workouts for women: 4 ways to build your back by design! Bodybuilding.Com. https://www.bodybuilding.com/content/back-workouts-for-women-4-ways-to-build-your-back-by-design.html

Cornish, J. L. (2020a, January 20). Arm workouts for women: 3 workouts to build size and strength. Bodybuilding.Com. https://www.bodybuilding.com/content/arms-workout-for-women-a-girls-guide-to-guns.html

Cornish, J. L. (2020b, March 11). The perfect partnership: Glute and hamstring workouts for women. Bodybuilding.Com. https://www.bodybuilding.com/content/glute-hamstrings-exercises-for-women-leg-workout.html

Creicos, B. (2016, July 30). Leg workouts for women: A girl's guide to glam gams. Bodybuilding.Com; Bodybuilding.com. https://www.bodybuilding.com/content/leg-workouts-for-women-a-girls-guide-to-glam-gams.html

DiDio, L. (2019, December 13). This workout tones and strengthens every inch of your body in just 15 minutes. Prevention. https://www.prevention.com/fitness/workouts/g25654172/15-minute-full-body-workout/

Eastman, H. (2017, November 7). The best workout for building massive quads. Bodybuilding.Com. https://www.bodybuilding.com/content/the-best-workout-for-building-massive-quads.html#:~:text=Leg%20Extension

Florio, G. (2018, May 26). 3 trainers explain exactly how to grow lean muscle and build curves. POPSUGAR Fitness. https://www.popsugar.com/fitness/Does-Lifting-Weights-Give-You-Curves-44338173

Geiger, B. (2015, September 16). 6 lessons that will transform your calves. Bodybuilding.Com. https://www.bodybuilding.com/content/6-lessons-that-will-transform-your-calves.html

Green, L. (2017, August 1). 7 strategies for conquering gym anxiety at any size. SELF. https://www.self.com/story/strategies-for-gym-anxiety-at-any-size

Halse, H. (2020, January 16). This beginner weight-lifting workout for women hits all your major muscles. LIVESTRONG.COM. https://www.livestrong.com/article/176944-beginning-weight-lifting-routine-for-women/

Harvard Health Publishing. (2019). Strength training builds more than muscles. Harvard Health; Harvard Health. https://www.health.harvard.edu/staying-healthy/strength-training-builds-more-than-muscles

Harvard T.H. Chan School of Public Health. (2012, September 18). Fats and cholesterol. The Nutrition Source. https://www.hsph.harvard.edu/nutritionsource/what-should-you-eat/fats-and-cholesterol/#:~:text=Fat%20is%20an%20important%20part

Jay. (2019, July 9). How to learn proper weight lifting form (and why it's so important). A Workout Routine. https://www.aworkoutroutine.com/proper-form/

Jha, A. (2017, December 28). How to build muscles fast at home without weights. YourStory.Com. https://yourstory.com/mystory/8f722f50f1-how-to-build-muscles-f

Kamb, S. (2019, January 21). How to build your own workout routine. Nerd Fitness. https://www.nerdfitness.com/blog/how-to-build-your-own-workout-routine/

Kelso, T. (n.d.). Butt-ology 101: How to enhance your gluteal muscles. Breaking Muscle. Retrieved July 8, 2020, from https://breakingmuscle.com/fitness/butt-ology-101-how-to-enhance-your-gluteal-muscles

Kerksick, C., Harvey, T., Stout, J., Campbell, B., Wilborn, C., Kreider, R., Kalman, D., Ziegenfuss, T., Lopez, H., Landis, J., Ivy, J. L., & Antonio, J. (2008). International society of sports nutrition position stand: Nutrient timing. Journal of the International Society of Sports Nutrition, 5(1). https://doi.org/10.1186/1550-2783-5-17

Leal, D. (2020, January 21). Good Food Choices to Eat After a Gym Workout. Verywell Fit. https://www.verywellfit.com/the-best-foods-to-eat-after-a-workout-3121369

Lexington Healing Arts Academy. (2019, April 3). Sixty five percent of women avoid the gym over a fear of being judged...Here's how to overcome this. Lexington Healing Arts Academy. https://www.lexingtonhealingarts.com/sixty-five-percent-of-women-avoid-the-gym-over-a-fear-of-being-judged-heres-how-to-overcome-this/

Pavlik Orthodontics. (2017, June 28). Top 7 benefits of self-confidence. Pavlik Orthodontics. http://pavlikortho.com/top-7-benefits-of-self-confidence/

Perine, S. (2020, April 16). Core killer! 6 workouts, 13 moves, 1 sculpted midsection! Bodybuilding.Com. https://www.bodybuilding.com/content/absolutely-perfect-abs-6-workouts-13-moves.html

Plosser, L. (2007, August 2). A WH fitness face off. Women's Health. https://www.womenshealthmag.com/fitness/a19921068/cardio-vs-strength-training-workouts/

Quinn, E. (2019, July 31). What and when to eat before exercising. Verywell Fit. https://www.verywellfit.com/what-to-eat-before-exercise-3120662

Reid, K. J., Baron, K. G., Lu, B., Naylor, E., Wolfe, L., & Zee, P. C. (2010). Aerobic exercise improves self-reported sleep and quality of life in older adults with insomnia. Sleep Medicine, 11(9), 934–940. https://doi.org/10.1016/j.sleep.2010.04.014

Rogers, P. (2019, March 10). What and when to eat for weight training. Verywell Fit. https://www.verywellfit.com/meal-timing-for-weight-training-3498426

Salomon WMN. (2020, May 5). The Radical Power of Challenging Yourself Outdoors. Outside Online. https://www.outsideonline.com/2411677/radical-power-challenging-yourself-outdoors#close

Schaefer, A. (2015, April 30). How many calories do you burn lifting weights? Healthline. https://www.healthline.com/health/fitness-exercise/calories-burned-lifting-weights#3

Semeco, A. (2016, September 20). Post-Workout nutrition: What to eat after a workout. Healthline; Healthline Media. https://www.healthline.com/nutrition/eat-after-workout#section1

Shaw, G. (2009, January 27). Women and weight training for osteoporosis. WebMD; WebMD. https://www.webmd.com/osteoporosis/features/weight-training#1

Sparacino, A. (2015, November 4). 25 genius ways fitness trainers stay motivated to exercise. Health.Com. https://www.health.com/weight-loss/25-genius-ways-fitness-trainers-stay-motivated-to-exercise

Stulberg, B. (2018, July 5). Battling Depression by Lifting Weights. Outside Online. https://www.outsideonline.com/2324201/lifting-weights-helps-ease-anxiety-and-depression#:~:text=The%20first%2C%20published%20in%202017

Unsplash. (n.d.-a). Photo by bruce mars on unsplash. Unsplash.-Com. Retrieved July 7, 2020, from https://unsplash.com/photos/WGN6ZEFEZbs

Unsplash. (n.d.-b). Photo by GMB monkey on unsplash. Unsplash.Com. Retrieved July 7, 2020, from https://unsplash.com/photos/ug_onUKP99Q

Unsplash. (n.d.-c). Photo by jonathan borba on unsplash. Unsplash.Com. Retrieved July 7, 2020, from https://unsplash.com/photos/lrQPTQs7nQQ

Unsplash. (n.d.-d). Photo by lindsey saenz on unsplash. Unsplash.Com. Retrieved July 7, 2020, from https://unsplash.com/photos/0cTbO9Swn2w

Unsplash. (n.d.-e). Photo by sergio pedemonte on unsplash. Unsplash.Com. Retrieved July 7, 2020, from https://unsplash.com/photos/K-DE9UZruLs

Unsplash. (n.d.-f). Photo by sergio pedemonte on unsplash. Unsplash.Com. Retrieved July 8, 2020, from https://unsplash.com/photos/1knFytoiXfI

Unsplash. (n.d.-g). Photo by Şule Makaroglu on unsplash. Unsplash.Com. Retrieved July 7, 2020, from https://unsplash.com/photos/YFmvjO3TP_s

Unsplash. (n.d.-h). Photo by sven mieke on unsplash. Unsplash.Com. Retrieved July 7, 2020, from https://unsplash.com/photos/jO6vBWX9h9Y

Women's Health. (2013, August 20). Your best body meal plan: Week 1. Women's Health. https://www.womenshealthmag. com/fitness/a19920774/six-week-weight-loss-plan-week-1/

Zaino, C. (2003, June 19). Consistency: The key to progress in your fitness program. Bodybuilding.Com. https://www. bodybuilding.com/fun/zaino16.htm